In memory of
Pamela Baldwin

STRESS IN HEALTH PROFESSIONALS

Psychological and Organisational Causes and Interventions

Edited by

Jenny Firth-Cozens
University of Northumbria at Newcastle, UK
and

Roy L. Payne
Curtin University of Technology, Western Australia

JOHN WILEY & SONS, LTD

Chichester · New York · Weinheim · Brisbane · Singapore · Toronto

Copyright © 1999 by John Wiley & Sons Ltd,
Baffins Lane, Chichester,
West Sussex PO19 1UD, England

National   01243 779777
International   (+44) 1243 779777
e-mail (for orders and customer service enquiries):
cs-books@wiley.co.uk
Visit our Home Page on http://www.wiley.co.uk
or http://www.wiley.com

Other Wiley Editorial Offices

John Wiley & Sons, Inc., 605 Third Avenue,
New York, NY 10158-0012, USA

WILEY-VCH Verlag GmbH, Pappelallee 3,
D-69469 Weinheim, Germany

Jacaranda Wiley Ltd, 33 Park Road, Milton,
Queensland 4064, Australia

John Wiley & Sons (Asia) Pte Ltd, 2 Clementi Loop #02-01,
Jin Xing Distripark, Singapore 129809

John Wiley & Sons (Canada) Ltd, 22 Worcester Road,
Rexdale, Ontario M9W 1L1, Canada

Library of Congress Cataloging-in-Publication Data

Stress in health professionals : psychological and organizational
  causes and interventions / edited by Jenny Firth-Cozens, Roy L.
  Payne.
        p.   cm.
    Includes bibliographical references and index.
    ISBN 0-471-99875-3 (cloth). — ISBN 0-471-99876-1 (paper : alk.
paper)
    1. Medical personnel—Job stress.   2. Medical personnel–
–Psychology.   3. Stress (Psychology)   I. Firth-Cozens, Jenny.
II. Payne, Roy.
    [DNLM: 1. Stress, Psychological.   2. Health Personnel.   WM 172
S915353   1999]
    R690.S785   1999
    155.9'042'08861—dc21
DNLM/DLC
for Library of Congress   99-29659
                                                              CIP

British Library Cataloguing in Publication Data

A catalogue record for this book is available from the British Library

ISBN 0-471-99875-3 (cloth)
ISBN 0-471-99876-1 (paper)

Typeset in 10/12pt Palatino by Dorwyn Ltd, Rowlands Castle, Hants
Printed and bound in Great Britain by Bookcraft (Bath) Ltd, Midsomer Norton, Somerset
This book is printed on acid-free paper responsibly manufactured from sustainable forestry, in which at least two trees are planted for each one used for paper production.

CONTENTS

Part III   Interventions for stress

ABOUT THE EDITORS

Jenny Firth-Cozens is Professor of Clinical Psychology at the University of Northumbria at Newcastle and Director of the Centre for Clinical Psychology and Health Care Research there. Her principal research interests and published works are in the field of occupational stress, particularly in health professionals; the influence of early experience on workplace dynamics; and organisational change in the context of improving the quality of patient care and reducing risk. She is both a clinical and occupational psychologist and enjoys working within the overlap of these fields. She was previously Principal Research Fellow at the University of Leeds and head of clinical effectiveness in the Northern and Yorkshire Region and has worked as a private organisational consultant, primarily in healthcare. She is a Fellow of the British Psychological Society and the Royal Society of Arts, Manufactures and Commerce.

Roy L. Payne graduated in Psychology at Liverpool University and spent two years postgraduate study in the MRC Unit for Occupational Aspects of Ageing. From there he joined the Aston group at the University of Aston in Birmingham, then followed Derek Pugh to the London Graduate School of Business Studies. Seventeen years after leaving there he went as Professor of Organisational Behaviour to Manchester Business School, having spent the intervening years at the MRC/ESRC Social and Applied Psychology Unit at Sheffield University. He returned to Sheffield in 1992 to a chair in Organisational Behaviour at Sheffield University Management School, and from June 1997 has been Professor of Organisational Psychology at Curtin University of Technology, Perth, W. Australia. His work at Aston led to publications on organisational structure and climate/culture in particular, and he has also published extensively in the occupational stress area. These remain active interests as well as more recent work on trust in organisations. He has done research and consulting for major organisations in both the public and the private sector.

ABOUT THE AUTHORS

Pamela Baldwin was formerly a lecturer in the University of Edinburgh with responsibilities for the medical undergraduate curriculum and training in Clinical Psychology. For the last few years she carried out and implemented research into the health, working conditions and training of NHS staff in the UK, and was awarded the 1998 BUPA Prize for research in the field of health and work. She died in May 1999.

Michael Barkham trained as a clinical psychologist and worked for ten years for the Medical Research Council undertaking trials of contrasting psychotherapies at the Social and Applied Psychology Unit at the University of Sheffield. Currently, he is involved in the development of the Clinical Outcomes in Routine Evaluation (CORE) system and has an abiding interest in the implementation of quality evaluation in service settings At present he is Senior Lecturer in Clinical Psychology and Head of the Psychological Therapies Research Centre in the School of Psychology at the University of Leeds.

Carol Borrill is an organisational psychologist with many years of research and consultancy experience in the National Health Service (NHS). She is based at Aston Business School, Aston University. She has just completed a large-scale research study on the prevalence and causes of stress among staff in the NHS, and evaluated interventions designed to reduce stress. She is currently involved in three research projects in the NHS: the effectiveness of team working in health care; the relationship between organisation, people management and trust performance and the relationship between team working and clinical effectiveness in breast cancer care teams.

Angela Carter has worked in the health service as a radiotherapy radiographer, teacher manager, and internal consultant and in the Institute of Work Psychology at the University of Sheffield conducting research on the prevalence of stress in the NHS. Her own PhD research is based in the context of the high strain environment of health care exploring whether it is better for people's well-being to work in a team or to work alone. Angela works as an independent occupational psychologist.

Cary L. Cooper is currently BUPA Professor of Organisational Psychology and Health in the Manchester School of Management, and Pro-Vice-Chancellor (External Activities) of the University of Manchester Institute of Science and Technology (UMIST). He is the author of over 80 books (on occupational stress, women at work and industrial and organisational psychology), has written over 300 scholarly articles for academic journals, and is a frequent contributor to national newspapers, TV and radio. He is currently Founding Editor of the *Journal of Organizational Behavior*, co-Editor of the medical journal *Stress Medicine*; co-Editor of the *International Journal of Management Review*. Professor Cooper is the Editor (jointly with Professor Chris Argyris of Harvard Business School) of the international scholarly *Blackwell Encyclopedia of Management* (12 volume set). He has been an adviser to the World Health Organisation, ILO, and recently published a major report for the EU's European Foundation for the Improvement of Living and Work Conditions on 'Stress Prevention in the Workplace'.

Tricia Cresswell is the Director of Public Health and Health Strategy for Newcastle and North Tyneside Health Authority. She has had involvement in child protection issues at several levels from membership of a local Area Child Protection Committee (when in general practice), to drafting national guidance. Her studies include a regional audit of health professional practice in child protection.

Robert Hale has been Director of the Portman Clinic since 1994, where he is also consultant psychiatrist in psychotherapy and psychoanalysis. He is a Fellow of the Royal College of Psychiatrists and Associate Dean, North Thames Postgraduate Medical and Dental Education with special responsibility for doctors in need of psychological help. His research interests are suicide, patients with AIDS, confidentiality, treating patients who suffer from sexual deviation or who display criminal behaviour, and the psychological needs of doctors.

Gillian Hardy is a clinical research fellow at the Psychological Therapies Research Centre, University of Leeds, and at the Institute of Work Psychology, University of Sheffield. She has been involved in a large study of stress within the health service in the UK. Her research interests cover stress at work and the outcomes and processes of psychological therapies. She has published widely in both these fields.

Clare Haynes has been working as an Occupational Psychologist researcher at the Institute of Work Psychology, University of Sheffield, since graduating from her MSc in 1993. She is currently project managing a 12-month management development programme with a grant awarded by the ESRC. Prior to this, she worked on the NHS Workforce Initiative, which was a Department of Health funded project with four main objectives: to examine the prevalence of stress among NHS staff; to determine the key work-related factors associated with stress; to determine the relationship between stress and absence/turnover; and to identify, and implement interventions to reduce stress.

Joe Herbert is reader in Neuroendocrinology in the Department of Anatomy at the University of Cambridge. His principal interests are stress and the brain, with particular reference to the chemical and genetic responses of the brain to demand, and the consequences this has for mental health, specifically major depressive disorder. His laboratory and clinical work is supported by grants from Wellcome Trust, MRC and BBSRC.

Larry Hirschhorn is a principal with the Center for Applied Research, a management consulting firm in Philadelphia. He has consulted to a broad range of organisations in the areas of strategy formulation and organisational development. He is recognised as an expert in the field of team dynamics, organisational development and change and the links between team dynamics and the strategy process. He has written several books— *Managing in the New Team Environment, The Workplace Within: Psychodynamics of Organizational Life* and (his most recent) *Reworking Authority: Leading and Following in the Post-Modern Organization*—and many articles on these subjects. Dr Hirschhorn is a founding member and past president of the International Society for Psychoanalytic Study of Organizations.

John Howie is Professor of General Practice at the University of Edinburgh and a principal in general practice. His research interests have included the determinants of decision making in general practice, and that led to the collaboration with Mike Porter that has underpinned the chapter in this book. He is now interested in the definition and delivery of quality of care at general practice consultations.

Liam Hudson was Professor of Psychology at Brunel University and Visiting Professor to the Tavistock and Portman Clinics in London. He has published widely in the field of work and relationships and in 1997 was invited to give the Tanner Lecture at Yale University. He and his wife, Bernadine Jacot, now run the Balas Copartnership, a consultancy practice in Buckinghamshire.

Linda May is a management consultant and anthropologist whose focus is helping clients in large, complex organisations bring about change. Dr

May is an associate at the Center for Applied Research, a Philadelphia-based management consulting firm that specialises in strategy, organisational effectiveness and market and industry analysis—with emphasis on the intersections among these practice areas. She is a core member of two of the research and development efforts at the Center: one R&D group is exploring new media in organisational life; the second is developing a "campaign" approach to organisational change. She joined the Center after serving as director of planning for the central computing division at the University of Pennsylvania.

Fiona Moss works both as a Consultant Physician in Respiratory Medicine at the Central Middlesex Hospital NHS Trust, London, and as an Associate Postgraduate Dean in North Thames with responsibility for Pre-Registration House Officer posts. She is working with colleagues in North Thames to develop better pre-registration training through better integration of the organisation of training and health care delivery, and new approaches to the structure of the pre-registration year. Prior to taking up her post as an Associate Postgraduate Dean she was a Consultant Physician within the Directorate of Public Health, North Thames, with responsibility for developing clinical audit. She is the Editor of the BMJ publishing group journal *Quality in Health Care*. Her current research interests include medical education and the quality of care.

Lawrence R. Murphy is senior research psychologist in the Division of Biomedical and Behavioral Science, National Institute for Occupational Safety and Health (NIOSH), and Associate Professor, Xavier University, Cincinnati, Ohio. He received his M.A. and Ph.D. degrees from DePaul University, Chicago, Illinois, and postdoctoral training at the Institute for Psychosomatic and Psychiatric Research, Michael Reese Medical Center. He has published numerous articles in the area of occupational stress and stress management, and co-edited several books, including *Stress Management in Work Settings* (1989), *Stress and Well-Being at Work (1992)*, and *Organizational Risk Factors for Job Stress* (1995). His current research involves identifying characteristics of healthy and productive work organisations.

Elisabeth Paice is Dean Director of Postgraduate Medical and Dental Education, North Thames. Her previous posts included Consultant Rheumatologist and Clinical Tutor at the Whittington Hospital. She has a long-standing interest in the problems of young doctors and has published research on training in the pre-registration house officer and senior house officer grades. She is a member of the Council of the National Association of Clinical Tutors, the Executive Council of the Association for the Study of Medical Education, and the Education Committee of the British Medical Association. She edits the Education section of *Hospital Medicine*.

Mike Porter is Senior Lecturer in Social Sciences at the Department of General Practice, University of Edinburgh. Following his work on stress on general practitioners with John Howie, he has focused more on issues to do with community care and is currently interested in the meaning of and opportunities for 'patient-centred care'.

Wilmar B. Schaufeli is full Professor for Clinical and Organisational Psychology at the Psychology Department of Utrecht University, The Netherlands. He worked in the areas of Clinical Psychology, and Work and Organisational Psychology at Groningen University and Nijmegen University, respectively. In addition to over one-hundred publications about unemployment, job stress, professional burnout, and absenteeism, he is actively involved in organisational consultancy and in psychotherapeutic treatment of burned-out employees. He is the European editor of the journal *Work and Stress*.

Paul E. Spector is a Professor of Industrial/Organizational Psychology at the University of South Florida in the USA. His research interests concern the impact of jobs on the behaviour and well-being of people, including counterproductive behaviour, job satisfaction, job stress, and withdrawal behaviour. At present he is an Associate Editor for *Journal of Occupational and Organizational Psychology*, and the Point/Counterpoint Editor for *Journal of Organizational Behavior*. In 1991 the Institute for Scientific Information listed him as one of the 50 highest impact authors in psychology world wide from 1986 to 1990.

Charles Vincent qualified as a clinical psychologist and worked in the NHS for a number of years. Since 1985 he has worked at University College London, where he is now Reader in Psychology, conducting research on the causes and consequences of adverse events in medicine. He currently directs the Clinical Risk Unit which provides training and carries out research on clinical risk management.

Michael West is Professor of Work and Organizational Psychology at the University of Aston Business School. He has been co-Director of the Corporate Performance Programme of the Centre for Economic Performance at the London School of Economics since 1991. He has authored, edited or co-edited 12 books, including *Developing Creativity in Organizations* (1997, BPS) and the *Handbook of Workgroup Psychology* (1996, Wiley). He has also written more than 120 articles for scientific and practitioner publications, and chapters in scholarly books. He is a fellow of the British Psychological Society, the American Psychological Association, the APA Society for Industrial/Organizational Psychology and the Royal Society for Arts, Manufactures and Commerce. His areas of research interest are team and organizational innovation and effectiveness.

Richard Whittington is a Senior Lecturer in the Department of Psychology, Chester College of Higher Education. He is a psychologist with a particular interest in workplace violence, especially violence to health care professionals, and previously worked as a psychiatric nurse in London. He has published research on individual and social factors associated with violence in mental health and general hospital settings and on post-assault stress among staff.

Til Wykes is a Reader in Clinical Psychology at the Institute of Psychiatry in London. She has varied research interests although the main focus of her attention has been on caring for people with schizophrenia. Her research has included both service evaluation, the effects of violence on staff and patients as well as the development of novel psychological treatments for people with schizophrenia. She was presented with the May Davidson Award in 1995 by the British Psychological Society for her contribution to the care of people with severe mental illness.

Kathryn Young is currently working in consultancy and retains links with the Manchester School of Management of the University of Manchester Institute of Science and Technology (UMIST). She has been involved in two studies focusing on the management of post-incident reactions in the workplace for the Health and Safety Executive (HSE). Her main research interests lie in the identification and management of traumatic stress in the workplace, especially in the emergency services.

PREFACE

The first edition of this book was published in 1987 at a time when there was a growing recognition that health workers were more stressed and experienced different stressors to other occupational groups. The research on this was relatively new with very few longitudinal studies and a focus on doctors in particular. Nevertheless, the chapters were able to outline the main issues and to set the stage for a research agenda that has progressed remarkably well over the intervening years.

The present edition reports much of this new research. Its chapters show that we are now able to describe the levels and sources of stress for most of the professionals involved in health care. Perhaps more important, this knowledge has led to the emphasis shifting towards interventions, both organisational and individual, and this has become an important part of this new edition.

Over the intervening years health services around the world have been subjected to a sharp escalation of change, and professionals have had to meet new demands and new conflicts as a result. Growing economic pressures, technological advances and patient expectations have meant that issues such as rationing, evidence-based health care, clinical audit and accreditation present staff with new demands and levels of accountability. Costs have become a crucial part of the agenda at every level while, at the same time, the quality of care delivered has become increasingly open to professional and public scrutiny.

However, the research has also shown that the stress levels of staff are intimately linked to both the cost and the quality of the care they deliver. Absence and turnover have long been associated with high stress levels, but now we also see disturbing deficits in recruitment in many professional groups: young doctors and nurses, for example, are leaving their professions in unprecedented numbers, despite the uncertainty of the job market outside of health care. The growth of early retirement, especially on the grounds of ill-health, also creates new pressures and expense to the service. Other rising costs involve the increase in litigation as patients' expectations rise along with their willingness to sue. As we know that high stress is linked to poorer performance, and that the vast proportion of accidents still escape scrutiny, there is a great need to tackle this area at once in a drive to reduce costs, as well as increasing the quality of life for health staff and patients alike. In addition to all this, stress is a health and safety issue which increasing numbers of staff in many public service posts are using as the foundation for legal action against their employers. The costs of stress are undoubtedly high and growing, and interventions to prevent and combat stress are essential.

This book uses contributions from the perspectives of occupational psychologists, clinicians (including doctors, psychoanalysts and psychologists), educationalists and physiologists. It begins with a general outline of occupational stress and the issues involved, and goes on to discuss the subject in terms of a number of specific professional groups within health care: doctors, nurses, managers, ambulance, workers, etc. The final section relates to key issues facing researchers within the field as well as those concerned with change: such areas as the impact of litigation and mistakes, individual differences, teamworking, burnout, the physiology of stress, and interventions. The means of bringing about organisational, team and individual interventions are described in new detail and range from ways to set up and evaluate counselling services, issues around training and team development, and case studies of work with individuals and with teams.

There is no doubt that recognition of the problem and progress in research in this field have been huge since 1987, and equally that this progress is continuing. The need now is to continue to develop ways to help impaired staff and their colleagues to recognise stress and other psychological problems more quickly and effectively, and to provide evidence-based interventions. Research over the next decade will undoubtedly be focusing on the evaluation of such interventions. It will also need to focus on the necessary change in the culture of health care from one in which stress is something that is borne by individuals to one in which it is seen as a barrier to the delivery of cost-effective quality care. Such a change in culture will require the collaboration of policy makers, management, unions, professional bodies and health workers from all levels of the health care system. The well-being of the workforce is a prerequisite to the well-being of the patient.

Jenny Firth-Cozens
10 January 1999

PART I

ISSUES IN STUDYING STRESS

1

STRESS AT WORK: A CONCEPTUAL FRAMEWORK

Roy Payne

The aim of this chapter is to introduce the reader to key concepts and frameworks in the literature on stress in the workplace. As I have indicated elsewhere (1995) there are at least three uses of the word, both in common parlance and in the academic literature. "Stress" is used to indicate that something is a *cause* of a person feeling they are stressed: e.g. the amount of work I have to do is making me ill. "Feeling ill" labels the psycho-physiological reactions which are the *consequence* of the large workload. Finally the word is used to describe the *process* which occurs when people find themselves unable to deal adequately with the demands made upon them. "The pressure builds up, I get tired and then anxious, and begin to make mistakes, which makes me more anxious, and I just want to run away, etc."

In this chapter I shall use the word stress in the general sense to refer to the *process* which involves some things which cause or precipitate individuals to think they are unable to cope with the situation that faces them, and the resulting feelings of anxiety, tension, frustration, anger which result from the recognition that they are failing in some way and the situation is getting out of their control. There is a tradition in industrial and organisational psychology of using the word *stressor(s)* to refer to the things that are causing these emotions, and the word *strain* to refer to the

Stress in Health Professionals. Edited by Jenny Firth-Cozens and Roy L. Payne
© 1999 John Wiley & Sons Ltd

consequences. This follows the way the terms stress and strain are used in engineering. In the medical literature, however, "stress" is used to refer to the outcome so we shall use the terms stressors and stress to refer to the causes and consquences, respectively.

Using "stress" to also refer to the process fits closely with the way it was defined by one of the pioneers of stress research, Hans Selye (1976). Selye was a doctor of medicine who became interested in the physiological and disease consequences of exposure to physical and emotional stressors. Selye concluded that when animals and humans are exposed to demands from the environment they respond with a broad pattern of physiological responses which, in humans, have associated emotional responses attached to them. The emotions vary in type and strength according to how well the demands are coped with. This pattern was called the General Adaptation Syndrome, or GAS for short.

The main events in this adaptive syndrome are that the digestion slows to release blood for muscles, and breathing increases to supply extra oxygen which causes the heart to accelerate, blood pressure to rise, and the muscles to prepare for action. If the muscles become highly active then perspiration increases to help cool the skin. These effects are largely under the control of the hormonal system and the major agents involved in the stress response are adrenaline, noradrenaline and cortisol, which have become widely used in studies of stress both in the laboratory and in the workplace (Fried, 1988). A more detailed explanation can be found in Tsigos and Chrousos (1996) and in Herbert's chapter in this book (Chapter 4).

If the actions taken are adequate to deal with the stressors then the GAS process will return the physiological and psychological systems to normal levels of functioning and little harm will have occurred either physiologically or psychologically. That is, the person has been exposed to an acute stressor but coped with it succcessfully, and so the stress disappears. The stressors may cease for some other reason of course (e.g. somebody else removes the stressor). The GAS becomes of relevance to the study of stress when the person's actions fail to cope with demands and they continue over lengthy periods of time. Selye describes the stages of the GAS as: *Alarm* in preparation to fight off the threat, run away from it or hide from it, followed by *Resistance* when the psycho-physiological system functions somewhat less actively and is striving to cope. If this period of resistance fails then the person ends up *Exhausted* because of the depletion of the body's stores of vitamins, sugars, proteins and immune defences. The exhaustion stage has become known in the literature as "burnout" (Maslach, 1982, and see Schaufeli's chapter in this book). It is these ongoing, chronic states that make stress medically interesting because of their relevance to both physical and psychological well-being.

This is not to say that some acute states of stress, or ones where the originating stressors don't last very long, do not also have severe consequences for health. Kleber and Van Der Velden (1996) describe the consequences of such acute stressors in the workplace showing how brief events such as being the victim of a robbery, or dealing with the casualties of bomb attacks, can develop into long lasting post-traumatic stress disorders. These sorts of events apart, however, the bulk of the literature on occupational stress has been concerned with jobs and situations where the stressors continue for some length of time, and what it is about the conditions in the workplace that lead to such stress, and their links to the possibility of damaging health and well-being. There is also concern on behalf of managers and owners to have a productive (healthy) workforce, which is strengthened in the current economic climate where there is a growing belief among Strategic Human Resource Managers and Chief Executive Officers that an organisation's people are its most valuable asset (e.g. Sparrow, 1994).

While it is useful, indeed necessary, to use stressors and stress to separate causes and consequences in the stress process, the word stressors does imply that more is worse. Both physiologically and psychologically this is not neccessarily the case. Not enough pressure on the body (exercise) causes it to deteriorate, and not enough stimulation in the environment leads to boredom, lethargy, deterioration of skills and withdrawal. Figure 1.1 combines the concepts of duration and strength of stressors to suggest the different psychological outcomes that are associated with different levels of each. A more elaborate and conceptually sophisticated version can be found in Payne (1982). As the figure shows, there is as much psychological stress from the combination of weak stressors/low pressure and long-term exposure to the situation, as there is from strong stressors/pressure and long-term exposure to that. Many unemployed, and some assembly line workers, face the first set of conditions and those who are "burnt-out" the second. The figure emphasises also that moderate amounts of pressure are required to stimulate and arouse people so that they perform to the maximum without crossing the line into high levels of stressors which last for medium to long periods of time. Stressful experiences of short to medium duration which are coped with effectively are often helpful, growth experiences in the long run as Maslow's work illustrates (Maslow, 1963). Maslow's self-actualisers are exceptional people perhaps, but the main purpose of Figure 1.1 is to illustrate the nature of situations that are stressful, and the variety of reactions to them, which include ones where some "stress" is actually beneficial.

A more detailed description of the process of stress is outlined in Figure 1.2. There are a number of frameworks similar to this one, but

	DURATION OF STRESSORS		
	Short term	Medium term	Long term
Weak Low demands	Bored Restless Lethargic	Torpidity Loss of direction Helplessness	Dismay Disillusionment Depression Sense of failure Alienation
Moderate Challenging demands	Aroused Liveliness Fun	Challenge Enjoyment Satisfaction Self-efficacy	Achievement Feelings of adequacy or competency and high self-esteem
Strong Excessive demands	High arousal Tension Excitement	Anger Fear Worry for future Tiredness Accomplishment (if coping)	Anxiety Depression Exhaustion Loss of self-confidence

STRENGTH OF STRESSORS

Figure 1.1: Some psychological outcomes of different stress situations

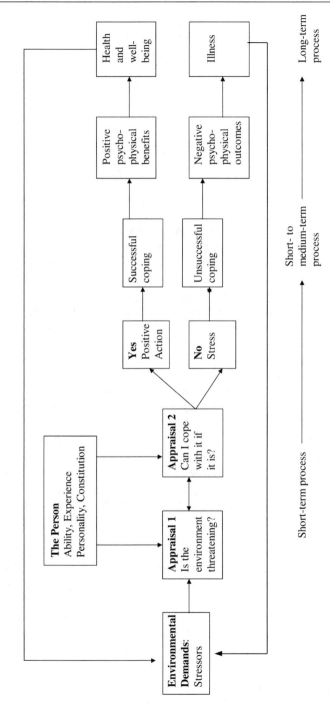

Figure 1.2: Stress as a process

this is heavily influenced by the work of Lazarus and Folkman (1984) who emphasised the importance of the person's role in appraising the situation which is what ultimately determines whether the situation is actually a stressor. For the masochist, being beaten is presumably a pleasure, and for the successful workaholic, another demanding task is merely a welcome challenge. Perception and cognition determine what the world means to us: one person's threat is another's opportunity.

As is hopefully evident from Figure 1.2, a person with certain abilities, experiences and personality is located in an environment which makes demands on him or her. Whether those demands constitute a stressor depends on the person's appraisal of whether they seem to be a threat, and if they are, the person faces the question, "Have I the ability, experience and character to meet these demands successfully?" If the answer is positive then, all things considered, the person tackles the demands with confidence and has a good chance of dealing with them successfully. If this occurs regularly then there are positive effects on physiological and psychological functioning and over the long term this leads to both good physical and psychological health. If people feel they cannot cope with the demands because they do not have the right abilities, experience and personality then the resulting stress leads to poorer problem-solving, which makes the problem worse. The feelings of failure, anxiety, and loss of confidence lead to negative physiological and psychological outcomes which over long periods affect both physical health and psychological well-being. These two inevitably influence each other, as the body of psychosomatic medical knowledge testifies. The feedback loops to such individuals are meant to indicate that these long-term effects can have an influence on their self-esteem, interpretation of themselves as people which will, in turn, influence their appraisal of similar situations in the future. All sorts of things can interrupt and change these processes of course, but this sort of framework is one that has guided researchers in trying to understand the effects of workplace stress.

Another way of illustrating this sort of framework is through what is called the Person–Environment "fit" model (French and Kahn, 1962). If the demands/stressors in the environment are matched by the person's knowledge, skills, abilities and needs then the person copes well with it and remains satisfied and healthy. The larger the misfit between the person's needs and abilities and the requirements of the job, for example, the greater the likelihood that he or she will be dissatisfied and stressed by it. Many people cope with highly stressful jobs because they have sought out an environment which "fits" them. This is true of many people in medicine and surgery.

THE ENVIRONMENT

One of the most enduring constructions of the work environment as stressor has been provided by Kahn *et al.* (1964). They used the social-psychological concept of role to analyse stress at work and developed measures of role conflict, role ambiguity, and role overload and showed that all three were associated with higher levels of psychological stress. In later studies of people from 23 different occupations colleagues from the same institute added other measures of stress, including physiological measures, and converted the concept of role overload to a much broader one called job demands (Caplan *et al.*, 1975). They found that it was not just the heaviness of the demands that led to stress. Occupations might have high demands and heavy responsibilities, but people in them might be less stressed because they have more control over their work, and more participation in decisions that affect them and the way they do their work. Indeed, if the working population (age 15–65 years) is categorised by social class, then death rates and morbidity rates for nearly all types of disease are lower for the higher social classes, many of whom have very demanding jobs. The high control and generous resources they usually have make the jobs less stressful (Fletcher, 1988). A few years after the work by Caplan *et al.* was published similar ideas, and further demonstrations of their empirical validity, were published in Karasek (1979).

Based on data from large samples in Sweden and the USA, Karasek showed that mental health, satisfaction at work, and satisfaction with life in general, are best predicted by a combination of two variables: job demands and level of decision latitude or discretion. Jobs which people perceived as high on demands and high on decision latitude (Active Jobs) produced high levels of satisfaction and positive mental health. This level of stress was originally termed "eustress" by Selye. What he termed "distress" is caused in Karasek's model by the combination of high demands and low decision latitude (High Strain Jobs). The combination of low demands and high discretion produces a relatively stress-free environment and people have lower stress and higher satisfaction (Low Strain Jobs). What Karasek called Passive Jobs are produced from the combination of low demands and low discretion and it is obvious enough that such jobs would be unlikely to provide great satisfaction which, in turn, is likely to lead to poorer psychological health.

A considerable amount of research has been generated from Karasek's ideas and this is well summarised in Jones and Fletcher (1996). They refer to studies which provide some support for the original model but many more which do not support the finding that it is the interaction between high demands and low discretion which produces the highest levels of strain. The studies do tend to show that discretion is the more important variable. The recognition of its importance led researchers to expand the concept to cover a range of things over which the worker could have discretion. In the process the concept became known as control, and Wall *et al.* (1996), for example, distinguish between timing control, method control and boundary control. They have shown how assembly line jobs with greater control led to higher output, satisfaction and fewer physical symptoms, but had no effect on mental health. Some writers on stress have seen control as so central to the idea that stress might well be defined as "being out of control of the situation". Jones and Fletcher (1996, p. 38) sum up the debate thus: "Overall, studies at the occupational level appear to provide evidence for the importance of control as a predictor of health outcomes, but less support for the demand–discretion interaction model."

At about the same time as Karasek's work appeared, another variable emerged as important in affecting how well people coped with stressful occupational environments. The variable is social support and Gore (1978) was one of the first to demonstrate its importance in dealing with the stress of unemployment. While it rapidly developed a literature of its own (e.g. House's book *Work, Stress and Social Support* was published in 1981) it was equally quickly absorbed into the demands–discretion framework. Payne (1979) published the Demands–Supports–Constraints model which proposed that all three concepts were multidimensional and thus superior to the simple demand and discretion variables proposed by Karasek, but that different combinations of the three would produce different psychological outcomes, more than one of which was "stressful". Different forms of psychological stress occur if the environment is low on demands, low on support and high on constraint (i.e. low control, tedious jobs) compared to high demands, high constraint and low support (stressful jobs). Modest support for the model was presented in Payne and Fletcher (1983) and Janman *et al.* (1988), but more importantly social support has continued to be an important variable in occupational stress research. Support now includes support from managers and supervisors, support from co-workers, support from family and friends, informational support and resource support. Jones and Fletcher (1996) review the evidence in relation to its addition to the demand–discretion model and conclude that ". . . social support is an important addition to the model, both because of the size of the main effects (much bigger than demands) and because some studies have found three-way interactions" (p. 42). That is, as outlined in the Payne model, stress is best predicted by the combination of high demands, low control and poor support. Indeed, lack of social support and the isolation associated with it is itself a stressor! The downsizing and continuous change that has bedevilled health care organisations in the last decade have made this a common occurrence in many branches of health care.

In later chapters it will be shown that hospital doctors have higher rates of stress than many other professions. In terms of the present model they would normally be seen as having high demands, but also high control derived from their professional status. But they have *very* demanding jobs in terms of hours worked and the responsibility they carry. Also, many junior doctors are quite controlled by their seniors and sometimes unsupported by them. Many hospital doctors have less control than one might think, and even very high levels of control might still not alleviate the effects of very high demands—wartime leaders are an extreme case, as are some chief executives and doctors.

In studying the work environment to see its effects on stress and satisfaction, it is important to examine the nature of the work demands, the control given to people dealing with the demands, and the support they receive from people, along with the support they receive in terms of resources. How these interact depends to some extent on the person faced with the situation, which brings us to the role of individual differences in the stress process depicted in Figure 1.2.

INDIVIDUAL DIFFERENCES

Individual differences arise from things which have largely been determined genetically such as gender and intellectual ability, from ascriptions we acquire as we develop, such as our age and social class, and from personality or dispositional factors which have developed under the influence of both our genes and our experience. Researchers have looked at differences in psychological and physical health for all these, and all have effects. Physical health and mental health both differ by social class, and thus by level in the organisation, with lower-class people tending to have poorer health and psychological well-being (Fletcher, 1988). Many young workers report higher levels of stress than more mature workers.

The largest area of interest, however, has been in personality or belief factors which affect how people react to stressful environments. Three prominent concepts have been Type A Behaviour, locus of control, and negative affectivity/trait anxiety. Type A Behaviour is a concept developed originally by two cardiologists to describe people they thought were more prone to suffer from coronary heart disease (Friedman and Rosenman, 1974). Type A individuals are those who behave in accordance with the pattern of striving to achieve, of meeting deadlines, walking and talking quickly and being hostile to people who interfere with their need to achieve and get things done. People who do not show these behaviours are Type B, and a huge body of research exists both in coronary heart disease, and because CHD is seen to be linked to stress, to stress research itself. The evidence in both fields is both positive and negative, but, on the whole, supportive in both. Type A individuals are more likely to seek out demanding situations, but to over-react to them and thus, in the long run, suffer more stress. A recent review relating Type A to health in general can be found in Rosenman (1996).

Locus of control is a concept construed by Rotter (1966) to account for differences in people's strength of beliefs about whether they are in control of the world or subject to control by the world. People who believe they are largely in control of what happens to them are described as being *Internals*, and those who believe they have little control of what happens (fatalistic) as being *Externals*. There is growing evidence that Externals are much more susceptible to becoming depressed (Presson and Benassi, 1996).

The third personality variable which is important in the stress field is negative affectivity, which is also measured by traditional personality questionnaires designed to measure trait anxiety or neuroticism (Watson and Clark, 1984). Such people see the world as a threatening place which, even when it might not be threatening, causes them to be anxious that it really is. It has become particularly important in self-report studies of work stress because it is argued that anxious people will see their environment as being full of stresors, that they will report higher levels of stress because of that, and these two effects bias the strength of the relationship between perceived demands and psychological stress. Brief *et al.* (1988) provided one of the first occupational examples of the effect and estimated the "true" relationship between perceived demands and reported stress by partialling out for the effect of negative affectivity. This practice has become widespread, and as the evidence has accumulated it has become clear that the strength of this moderating effect varies from zero to very strong, and Spector *et al.* (1998) have begun to question whether this partialling procedure is sensible. The relevance of negative affectivity, and now a growing interest in the effects of positive affectivity in the workplace (Watson and Pennebaker, 1989), remains undiminished, but it is very clear that understanding stress at work involves understanding the role of negative affectivity. Individual differences are dealt with more fully in the chapter by Spector.

Finally, it is important to include the idea of coping styles as individual difference variables. As is clear from Figure 1.2, having appraised the situation as threatening the person has to decide if their coping resources are able to deal with the threat. It has been argued (Lazarus and Folkman, 1984) that individuals differ in their habitual styles of coping so that some prefer a Problem-focused style and others an

Emotion-focused style, and other writers have developed measures of other styles (e.g. Moos, 1990). The Emotion-focused style relies on cognitive efforts to reinterpet the situation in some way (denial, rationalisation) and there is some evidence that it is less effective in coping with work-related problems in particular (Anderson, 1977), though it should be said the atempt to measure coping styles has proved much more difficult than originally imagined. Having briefly introduced the concepts of environmental stressors and individual differences which influence reactions to them, it remains to describe indicators of psychological and physiological stress themselves.

PSYCHO-PHYSIOLOGICAL INDICATORS OF STRESS

One way to categorise these is to distinguish between symptoms, thinking, behaving and feeling.

Symptoms

These include physiological indicators such as heart rate, blood pressure, and a range of hormones, the commonest of which are adrenaline, noradrenaline and cortisol which can be collected from saliva, urine and blood. They also include symptoms which occur frequenly among stressed people such as headaches, backaches, sweating, nausea, loss of control over bladder and bowels, and raised, possibly uneven, breathing patterns.

Thinking

In the extreme these might include paranoid thinking, but more common signs are forgetting, illogical thinking, irrational thinking, confused thinking, slowness of thinking and fixation of thinking so that creative problem solving is minimised. They also include thinking of yourself as worthless, and thinking of the world as incapable of influence by you, resulting in thinking oneself into hopelessness.

Behaving

The classic stress actions are, of course, fight, flight and freeze. In work situations these translate into aggressive behaviour/harassment, withdrawal from work by absence or resignation, or by doing all one can to avoid being noticed by anyone. Other actions which can be used to indicate the presence of stress are increases in the use of drugs such as alcohol, tobacco, tranquillisers and stimulants. It ought to be recognised that *change in use* is important here, and could even include decreases in use. As nicotine and alcohol are so common in western societies it cannot be concluded that even high usage means that the person is stressed. Indeed, for managers and concerned colleagues it is *changes in behaviour* that provide the best clues to the presence of stress in others. Unless they are extreme, symptoms, thinking processes and feelings can often be hidden by the stressed person.

Feelings

These include all the various degrees of, or synonyms for anxiety—tension, worry, panic, fear—but also other strong emotions such as anger, hopelessness, guilt and depression. Feelings are probably the first and the most powerful indicators of the presence of stress, but are so intimately connected to cognitive appraisals of the environment that they are inevitably and intimately involved in the stress process. As the process is prolonged they may turn into relatively enduring mood states as described in clinical descriptions of anxiety and depression.

CONCLUSION

This chapter has offered a framework for understanding stress at work which attempts to recognise that it is a process which takes place over different time periods, from very short periods lasting minutes, to very long ones lasting months or years. In doing so the framework tries to identify the main types of variables that are relevant to these different time periods, and the differing consequences of each. There is evidence to show that the work environment creates stressors, that the amount of stress is affected by the nature of the person who is exposed to it, and that the effects of stressors can be reduced by strategies such as increasing the control people have, and by increasing the kind of social supports available. It is also obvious that people can be trained and educated to adopt more effective coping strategies/styles. If stressors last for lengthy periods of time they have consequences for the long-term health and well-being of the workers exposed to them. While these claims are broadly supported by the empirical findings, the chapter has also indicated that the strength of the relationships between the variables varies across studies, and that the complexity of the stress process provides a considerable challenge to people studying it. Hopefully, this broad introduction will help to place the more specific chapters to follow in a useful intellectual context.

REFERENCES

Anderson, C.R. (1977). Locus of control, coping behaviours and performance in a stress setting: a longitudinal study. *Journal of Applied Psychology*, **62**, 44–51.

Brief, A.P., Burke, M.J., George, J.M., Robinson, B. and Webster, J. (1988). Should negative affectivity remain an unmeasured variable in the study of job stress? *Journal of Applied Psychology*, **73**, 193–198.

Caplan, R.D., Cobb, S., French, J.R.P., Harrison, R, van and Pinneau, S.R. (1975). *Job Demands and Worker Health*. Washington: National Institute for Occupational Safety and Health.

Fletcher, B. (C), (1988). The epidemiology of stress. In Cooper, C.L. and Payne R. (eds) *Causes, Coping, and Consequences of Stress at Work*. Chichester: Wiley.

French, J.R.P. Jr and Kahn, R.L. (1962). A programmatic approach to studying the industrial environment and mental health. *Journal of Social Issues*, **18**(3), 1–47.

Fried, Y. (1988). The future of physiological assessments in work situations. In Cooper, C.L. and Payne, R. (eds). *Causes, Copying, and Consequences of Stress at Work*. Chichester: Wiley.

Fried, Y., Rowland, K.M. and Ferris, G.R. (1984). The physiological measurement of work stress: a critique. *Personnel Psychology*, **37**, 583–615.

Friedman, M. and Rosenman, R.H. (1974). *Type A Behaviour and Your Heart*. London: Wildwood House.

Gore, S. (1978). The effect of social support in moderating the health consequences of unemployment. *Journal of Health and Social Behavior*, **19**, 157–165.

House, J.S. (1981). *Work, Stress and Social Support*. Reading, Mass.: Addison-Wesley.

Janman, K., Jones, G.J., Payne, R.L. and Rick, J.T. (1988). Clustering individuals as a way of dealing with multiple indicators in occupational stress research. *Behavioral Medicine*, Spring, 17–29.

Jones, F. and Fletcher, B.(C). (1996) Job control and health. In M.J. Shabracq, J.A.M. Winnibust and C.L. Cooper (Eds) *Handbook of Work and Health Psychology*. Chichester: Wiley.

Kahn, R.L., Wolfe, D., Quinn, R. and Snoek, J. (1964). *Organizational Stress: Studies in Role Conflict and Ambiguity*. New York: Wiley.

Karasek, R.A. (1979). Job demands, job decision latitude and mental strain: implications for job design. *Administrative Science Quarterly*, **24**, 285–308.

Kleber, R.J. and Van Der Velden, P.G. (1996). Acute stress at work. In M.J. Shabracq, J.A.M. Winnibust and C.L. Cooper (Eds) *Handbook of Work and Health Psychology*. Chichester: Wiley.

Maddi, S.R. and Kobassa, S.C. (1984). *The Hardy Executive: Health Under Stress*. Homewood, Ill.: Dow-Jones-Irwin.

Lazarus, R. and Folkman, S. (1984). *Stress, Appraisal and Coping*. New York: Springer.

Maslach, C. (1982). *Burnout: the Cost of Caring*. Englewood Cliffs, NJ: Prentice-Hall.

Maslow, A.H. (1963). *Towards a Psychology of Being*. Van Nostrand.

Moos, R.H. (1990). *Coping Responses Inventory Manual*. Dept of Psychiatry and Behavioral Sciences, Stanford University, Palo Alto, Ca.

Payne, R.L. (1979). Demands, supports, constraints and psychological health. In Mackay, C. and Cox, T. (Eds) *Response to Stress: Occupational Aspects*. London: IPC.

Payne, R.L. (1981). Stress in task focussed groups. *Small Group Research*, **12**(3), 253–268.

Payne, R.L. (1982). Stress and cognition in organizations. In D.V. Hamilton (Ed.) *Human Stress and Cognition*. Chichester: Wiley.

Payne, R.L. (1995). Stress. In N. Nicholson (Ed.) *Encylopedic Dictionary of Organizational Behaviour*. Oxford: Blackwell.

Payne, R.L. and Fletcher, B. (C). (1983). Job demands, supports and constraints as predictors of psychological strain among schoolteachers. *Journal of Vocational Behavior*, **22**, 136–147.

Presson, P.K. and Benassi, V.A. (1996). Locus of control orientation and depressive symptomology: a meta analysis. *Journal of Social Behaviour and Personality*, **11**(1), 201–212.

Rotter, J.B. (1966). Generalized expectancies for internal vs. external control of reinforcement. *Psychological Monographs*, **80**(1), Whole No. 609.

Rosenman. R.H. (1996). Personality, behaviour patterns and heart disease. In C.L. Cooper (ed.) *Handbook of Stress, Medicine, and Health*. Baton Roca, Fla: CRC Press.

Selye, H. (1976). *The Stress of Life*. New York: McGraw Hill.

Sparrow, P. (1994). The psychology of strategic management: emerging themes of diversity and cognition. In C.L. Cooper and I.T. Robertson (Eds) *International Review of Industrial and Organizational Psychology*, vol. 9. Chichester: Wiley.

Spector, P.E., Zapf, D., Chen, P.Y. and Frese, M. (1998). Why negative affectivity should not be controlled in job stress research: don't throw out the baby with the bath water. *Journal of Organizational Behaviour* (to appear).

Tsigos, C. and Chrousos, G.P. (1996). Stress, endocrine manifestations and diseases. In C.L. Cooper (Ed.) *Handbook of Stress, Medicine, and Health*. Baton Roca, Fla.: CRC Press.

Wall, T.D., Jackson, P.R., Mullarkey, S. and Parker, S.K. (1996). The demands-control model of job strain: a more specific test. *Journal of Occupational and Organizational Psychology*, **69**, 153–166.

Watson, D. and Clark, L.A. (1984). Negative affectivity: the disposition to experience aversive emotional states. *Psychological Bulletin*, **96**, 465–490.

Watson, D. and Pennebaker, J.W. (1989). Health complaints, stress and distress: exploring the central role of negative affectivity. *Psychological Review*, **96**, 234–254.

2

BURNOUT

Wilmar Schaufeli

INTRODUCTION

Burnout is a metaphor that describes a state of exhaustion, similar to the smothering of a fire or the extinguishing of a candle. The dictionary defines "to burn out" as: "to fail, wear out, or become exhausted by making excessive demands on energy, strength, or resources". Burnout was first described in greater detail by Herbert Freudenberger although occasional accounts of burnout *avant-la-lettre* had appeared before, not only in works of fiction but also in journals for professionals. As a psychiatrist, he observed that volunteers who worked with drug addicts experienced a gradual energy depletion and loss of motivation and commitment, which was accompanied by a wide array of other mental and physical symptoms. Freudenberger labelled this particular state of exhaustion "burnout": a colloquial term used to refer to the devastating effects of chronic drug abuse. Independently, and at about the same time, Christina Maslach—a social psychological researcher—stumbled across that very term in California (*cf.* Maslach and Schaufeli, 1993). She studied the ways in which health care professionals cope with emotional arousal at work and observed that many professionals were emotionally exhausted, had developed negative perceptions about their patients, and experienced a crisis in their professional competence.

Almost immediately after its discovery, burnout became a very popular topic, first in the popular press and then in academia. To date, more than 5,500 publications on the subject have appeared and over 1,000 empirical

Stress in Health Professionals. Edited by Jenny Firth-Cozens and Roy L. Payne
© 1999 John Wiley & Sons Ltd

studies were carried out, predominantly in health care (34%) and teaching (27%) (Schaufeli and Enzmann, 1998, pp. 69–73).

Three conclusions can be drawn from the history of burnout. First, burnout emerged as a social problem and *not* as a scholarly construct—it was "in the air", so to speak. Second, from the outset burnout was strongly associated with "people work" in the human services. Third, two different approaches to burnout developed and coexist more or less independently: a clinical approach initiated by Freudenberger and a research approach initiated by Maslach.

The purpose of this chapter is to present a comprehensive overview of burnout in health care. In the following sections attention is paid to (1) symptoms and assessment; (2) burnout, stress and depression; (3) the prevalence of burnout in health care; (4) correlates, causes and consequences; and (5) psychological explanations.

SYMPTOMS AND ASSESSMENT

Particularly in the initial pioneering phase when the clinical approach to burnout prevailed, many symptoms of burnout were identified. Recently, Schaufeli and Enzmann (1998, pp. 20–31) listed over 130 possible symptoms that have been associated with burnout, ranging from *a* (anxiety) to *z* (lack of zeal). Five symptom-clusters may be distinguished: (1) affective (e.g. depressed mood, emotional exhaustion); (2) cognitive (e.g. poor concentration); (3) physical (e.g. headaches, sleep disturbances); (4) behavioural (e.g. poor work performance); (5) motivational (e.g. loss of idealism). It is quite remarkable that—except for motivational symptoms—these clusters seem to match perfectly with the usual categorisation of stress symptoms. Typically, burnout is not restricted to symptoms at the individual level, in addition interpersonal symptoms in relation to recipients are also observed (e.g. irritability, dehumanisation, indifference) as well as symptoms at the organisational level (e.g. job dissatisfaction, job turnover, low morale).

However, such a laundry-list approach is inappropriate to define the syndrome since it denies that burnout is a process and it confuses symptoms with precursors, correlates and consequences. Instead, Schaufeli and Enzmann (1998, p. 36) reviewed various definitions of burnout and propose the following synthetic definition:

> *Burnout is a persistent, negative, work-related state of mind in "normal" individuals that is primarily characterised by exhaustion, which is accompanied by distress, a sense of reduced effectiveness, decreased motivation, and the development of dysfunctional attitudes and*

behaviours at work. This psychological condition develops gradually but may remain unnoticed for a long time for the individual involved. It results from a misfit between intentions and reality at the job. Often burnout is self-perpetuating because of inadequate coping strategies that are associated with the syndrome.

More specifically, this definition narrows down over one hundred burnout symptoms to one core indicator (exhaustion) and four accompanying, general symptoms: (1) distress (affective, cognitive, physical, and behavioural); (2) a sense of reduced effectiveness; (3) decreased motivation; (4) dysfunctional attitudes and behaviours at work. Furthermore, frustrated intentions and inadequate coping strategies play a role as preconditions in the development of burnout and the process is considered to be self-perpetuating despite the fact that it may not be recognised initially. Finally, the domain is specified: the symptoms are work-related and burnout occurs in "normal" individuals who do not suffer from psychopathology.

This description is somewhat more comprehensive than the probably most often cited definition:

Burnout is a syndrome of emotional exhaustion, depersonalisation, and reduced personal accomplishment that can occur among individuals who work with people in some capacity. (Maslach *et al.*, 1996, p. 4)

Its popularity is due to the fact that the most widely used self-report questionnaire—the Maslach Burnout Inventory (MBI)—comprises the three dimensions that are included in this definition. Emotional exhaustion refers to the depletion or draining of emotional resources. Depersonalisation points to the development of negative, callous, indifferent, and cynical attitudes toward the recipients of one's services. The term depersonalisation may cause some confusion since in psychiatry it denotes a person's extreme alienation from the self and from the world. In contrast, in Maslach *et al.*'s definition, depersonalisation refers to an impersonal and dehumanised perception of *recipients*. Finally, lack of personal accomplishment is the tendency to evaluate one's work with recipients negatively. It is believed that the objectives are not achieved, which is accompanied by feelings of insufficiency and poor professional self-esteem.

Because the MBI is *the* instrument to measure burnout, the definition of burnout has become equivalent with the way it is measured—burnout is what the MBI measures. This tautology seriously hampers burnout research since the concept of burnout—as previously defined—is broader and more comprehensive than the MBI assumes. On the other hand, because of this common standard, findings from different studies can be compared straightforwardly.

Generally speaking, the psychometric quality of the MBI is satisfactory (Schaufeli *et al.*, 1993). More specifically, the factorial validity and the convergent validity as well as the reliability of the MBI are quite encouraging. However, emotional exhaustion in particular overlaps with related concepts such as depression and job dissatisfaction, as well as with distress symptoms (see later). It seems that the most robust and reliable subscale—emotional exhaustion—that also displays the strongest convergent validity with other burnout measures, is at the same time the least specific dimension of burnout.

BURNOUT, STRESS AND DEPRESSION

Burnout has been equated with a myriad of terms, most of them are plagued by the same sort of definitional ambiguity. The most prominent examples are stress and depression. In what ways can burnout be distinguished from these two related concepts?

Stress is a generic term that refers to the temporary adaptation process that is accompanied by mental and physical symptoms. In contrast, burnout can be considered as a final stage in a breakdown in adaptation that results from the long-term imbalance of demands and resources. In other words, burnout results from prolonged job stress. Moreover, burnout includes the development of dysfunctional attitudes and behaviours towards recipients (depersonalisation), the job, and the organisation, whereas job stress is not necessarily accompanied by such attitudes and behaviours. This assertion is empirically supported by Schaufeli and Van Dierendonck (1993), who showed in a sample of nurses that MBI-burnout can be distinguished from generic job-related mental and physical distress, albeit emotional exhaustion shared about 30% of its variance with distress. Finally, it has been claimed that everybody can experience stress, while burnout can only be experienced by those who entered their careers enthusiastically with high goals and expectations. For example, Pines (1993) has argued that individuals who expect to derive a sense of significance from their work are susceptible to burnout, whereas those without such expectations would experience job stress instead of burnout.

Clearly, burnout and depression are characterised by similar dysphoric symptoms. Nevertheless, clinical practice suggests that both syndromes differ: depressive patients are generally overwhelmed by listlessness and lethargy and hold steadfastly to their ideas of guilt, whereas burnout victims present their complaints much more vigorously—they feel disappointed and aggrieved. Furthermore, contrary to depression, burnout tends to be job-related and situation-specific rather than pervasive, at least initially, affecting all other spheres of life. Finally, burnout includes specific dysfunctional attitudes and behaviours that are not typically found in depression. Recently, Glass and McKnight (1996) concluded after reviewing nearly twenty studies on burnout and depression: "Burnout and depressive symptomatology are not simply two terms for the same dysphoric state. They do, indeed, share appreciable variance (about 25%, W.S.), especially when the emotional exhaustion component is involved, but the results do not indicate complete isomorphism. We conclude, therefore, that burnout and depressive symptomatology are not redundant concepts" (p. 33).

Thus it seems that burnout can be distinguished conceptually as well as empirically from job stress and from depression. Nevertheless, emotional exhaustion shows some overlap with both concepts, which illustrates that this dimension resembles most closely a rather general and orthodox stress variable. The fact that depersonalisation and reduced personal accomplishment are less substantively related to the other concepts implies that burnout is a unique, multidimensional, chronic stress reaction that goes beyond the experience of mere exhaustion.

THE PREVALANCE OF BURNOUT IN HEALTH CARE

How often does burnout occur in health care? In principle, the MBI can be used to answer this question, but the distinction it makes between "cases" and "non-cases" is based on arbitrary statistical norms instead of norms that are clinically validated. Hence, the absolute prevalence of burnout in health care cannot be assessed; but what about relative levels of burnout? Table 2.1 presents an overview of mean MBI-scores across four occupational fields.

Levels of emotional exhaustion in health care (medicine and mental health) are relatively low, particularly when compared with teaching. Although levels of depersonalisation in health care are also relatively low, particularly when compared with the social services, physicians exhibit the highest scores. Finally, reduced personal accomplishment is least experienced in mental health care, particularly by psychologists and counsellors. Physicians also exhibit relatively low scores on this burnout dimension. Obviously, academically trained health professionals such as psychologists and physicians experience the highest levels of accomplishment in their jobs. Table 2.1 shows remarkable differences between professionals in both health care fields. Compared to physicians, nurses experience slightly less emotional exhaustion, but much less depersonalisation and personal accomplishment. Although gender bias cannot

Table 2.1:   Burnout levels across occupational fields: mean MBI-scores of 43 USA studies published between 1979 and 1998

Occupational field Profession	Samples		Emotional exhaustion		Depersonal- isation		Reduced personal accomplishment	
	No.	N	Mean	SD	Mean	SD	Mean	SD
Teaching	6	5,481	28.15	11.99	8.68	6.46	11.65	7.41
Social services	7	1,631	24.29	12.79	9.47	7.16	13.45	8.55
Medicine	14	2,021	23.86	11.57	7.95	6.47	12.38	7.96
Nurses	11	1,542	23.80	11.80	7.13	6.25	13.53	8.15
Physicians	3	479	24.03	10.77	10.59	6.46	8.64	5.93
Mental health	12	2,137	20.27	9.81	6.22	4.54	8.81	6.46
psychologists/ counsellors	6	1,804	19.93	9.59	6.26	4.41	8.36	6.23
Staff	6	333	22.09	10.96	6.03	5.22	11.24	7.58
Total	39	11,270	25.33	11.65	8.19	6.26	11.50	7.52

Note: Adapted from Schaufeli and Enzmann (1998, p. 62).

be ruled out—nurses are predominantly female and females tend to report less depersonalisation than males (Schaufeli and Enzmann, 1998, p. 76)—it is likely that differences in depersonalisation reflect different professional roles and attitudes: the nurturing and caring role of the nurse versus the more distant curing role of the doctor. In mental health care non-academic staff experience more emotional exhaustion and less accomplishment than psychologists and counsellors. Probably this reflects the more stressful nature of the jobs of the former that are characterised by less decision latitude (perhaps leading to emotional exhaustion), as well as their less extensive training (perhaps leading to a sense of reduced personal accomplishment).

CORRELATES, CAUSES AND CONSEQUENCES

Despite the impressive quantity of empirical publications on burnout, their quality is often questionable. Accordingly, results have to be interpreted with caution. Table 2.2 summarises the most important correlates of burnout that are found in health care (*cf.* Cordes and Dougherty, 1993; Lee and Ashforth, 1996; Schaufeli and Enzmann, 1998, pp. 69–99).

Biographical characteristics   Among younger employees burnout is observed more often than among those aged over 30 or 40 years. This is in line with the observation that burnout is negatively related to work

Table 2.2: Correlates of burnout in health care

Biographic characteristics	Young age Little work experience
Personality	Less "hardy" personality External locus of control Poor self-esteem Non-confronting coping style Neuroticism "Feeling type"
Work-related attitudes	High (unrealistic) expectations Job dissatisfaction Poor organisational commitment Intention to quit
General job stressors	High workload Time pressure Role conflict and ambiguity Lack of social support Lack of feedback Lack of participation in decision making Lack of autonomy
Specific job stressors	Much direct patient contact Severe patient problems
Individual health	Depression Psychosomatic complaints Frequency of illness
Organisational behaviour	Absenteeism Job turnover Impaired performance

experience. The greater incidence of burnout among the younger and less experienced may be caused by "reality shock" or by an identity crisis due to unsuccessful occupational socialisation. However, a cautionary note should be made because survival bias cannot be ruled out: those who burn out early in their careers are likely to quit their jobs, leaving behind the survivors, who exhibit low levels of burnout (see later).

Personality   Burnout is less common among those with a "hardy person-ality" who are characterised by involvement in daily activities, a sense of control over events, and openness to change. In contrast, burnout is more common among those with an external "locus of control" who attribute events and achievements to powerful others or to chance compared to those with an internal locus, who ascribe events and achievements to their own ability, effort, or willingness to risk. Moreover, burnout is related to poor self-esteem and an avoidant, non-confronting coping style.

Burnout seems to be particularly related to neuroticism. Typically, emotional exhaustion shares about 30% of its variance with neuroticism, and 10–15% with the remaining factors. Depersonalisation and reduced personal accomplishment share about 5–10% of their variance with personality factors, with the latter being somewhat more strongly related to an avoiding coping style (15%) (Schaufeli and Enzmann, 1998, pp. 77–80). Since neurotic individuals are emotionally unstable and prone to psychological distress, neuroticism may act as a vulnerability factor that predisposes professionals to experience burnout.

Finally, compared to "thinking types", "feeling types" are more prone to burnout, especially to depersonalisation (Garden, 1991). The former are more hard-boiled, achievement-oriented and tend to neglect others, whereas the latter are more tender-minded and are characterised by concern and awareness for people. According to Garden (1991), "feeling types" are over-represented in health care and "thinking types" are more often found in business, which might explain the relatively high prevalence of burnout in the former sector.

Work-related attitudes Although high and unrealistic expectations are related to burnout, this association is not as strong and unequivocal as might be expected. This is probably caused by the fact that different concepts are used, such as omnipotence, irrational beliefs, idealism, unmet expectations, disillusionment, and outcome expectations. Furthermore, it is not always clear whether expectations refer to the organisation, to patients' progress, or to personal effectiveness. Job dissatisfaction, poor organisational commitment, and intention to quit—all indicators of psychological withdrawal—share considerable amounts of variance with burnout: 5–25%, depending on the dimension involved (Schaufeli and Enzmann, 1998, p. 80). The strongest associations are found with emotional exhaustion and depersonalisation.

General job stressors Workload and time pressure explain about 25 to 50% of variance of burnout, especially of emotional exhaustion (see Lee and Ashforth, 1996). Relationships are much weaker with both other MBI-dimensions. The high correlation with workload must be qualified, however, because this stressor is often operationalised in terms of experienced strain so that considerable overlap in item content exists with emotional exhaustion. On the other hand, Intensive Care Units' use of technology—objectively assessed by the number of patients who were mechanically ventilated—was substantively related to nurses' burnout levels (Schaufeli, *et al.*, 1995).

Role conflict (i.e. conflicting demands at the job have to be met) and role ambiguity (i.e. no adequate information is available to do the job well) are moderately to highly correlated with burnout. Role conflict shares about 24% of variance with emotional exhaustion, 13% with depersonalisation, and only 2% with personal accomplishment; the percentages for role ambiguity are 14, 8, and 10% respectively (Schaufeli and Enzmann, 1998, pp. 82–83).

Clear evidence exists for a positive relationship between lack of social support and burnout, especially lack of social support from supervisors. On the average, support from supervisors explains 14% of the variance of emotional exhaustion, 6% of depersonalisation, and 2% of personal accomplishment; for co-workers the amounts of variance are 5, 5 and 2% respectively (see Lee and Ashforth, 1996). The longitudinal study of Leiter and Durup (1996) among health care professionals showed that emotional exhaustion predicted work overload and supervisor support, instead of the other way round, suggesting a cyclical process rather than straight causation.

Finally, three factors that determine self-regulation of work activities are related to burnout: lack of feedback, poor participation in decision making, and lack of autonomy (Landsbergis, 1988).

Specific job stressors   Recently Schaufeli and Enzmann (1998, pp. 84–85) compared the results of 16 studies and found that, overall and contrary to expectations, common job-related stressors such as workload, time pressure, or role conflicts correlate more highly with burnout than do patient-related stressors such as interaction with difficult patients, problems in interacting with patients, frequency of contact with chronically or terminally ill patients, or confrontation with death and dying. For instance, Mallett *et al.* (1991) found among nurses only weak correlations between the death of patients and emotional exhaustion and depersonalisation. Instead, lack of staffing and insufficiently qualified staff were considered the most stressful aspects of their work. Obviously, confrontation with death and dying of patients is not the most disturbing part of the nurses' job. It is likely that nurses have developed adaptive mechanisms to these which prevent negative long-term effects such as burnout.

Individual health   Significant correlations with self-report measures of depression and psychosomatic distress are often reported (Schaufeli and Enzmann, 1998, pp. 86–89). As noted above, burnout cannot be reduced to mere depressed mood or distress, yet it is related to both conditions.

As far as self-reported frequency of various illnesses is concerned, Corrigan *et al.* (1995) reported among psychiatric hospital staff a shared variance with emotional exhaustion plus depersonalisation of 18%. In a similar vein, Landsbergis (1988) found a significant positive relationship between nurses' self-reported symptoms of coronary heart disease and emotional exhaustion (3% shared variance) and depersonalisation (4%); the relationship with reduced personal accomplishment was not significant (2%).

Organisational behaviour   Despite the popular assumption that burnout causes absenteeism, its effect is rather small and is best confirmed with respect to emotional exhaustion and next by depersonalisation. On average, about 2% of variance is shared with registered absenteeism; relations with reduced personal accomplishment are marginal but significant (Schaufeli and Enzmann, 1998, pp. 91–92).

Levels of depersonalisation predict nurses' actual job turnover within two years (Firth and Britton, 1989), whereas levels of emotional exhaustion predict turnover among general practitioners within five years (Sixma *et al.*, 1998). In terms of shared variance, the significant effects are rather low, ranging between 1 and 5%. The fact that the relationship of burnout with turnover intentions is much stronger than with actual turnover, suggests that a large percentage of burned out professionals stay in their jobs reluctantly.

It is important to distinguish between self-ratings of performance and objective measures or ratings by others such as co-workers or supervisors. Self-rated performance correlates weakly with burnout; roughly 5% of variance is shared with all three MBI-dimensions against less than 1% for other-rated or objectively assessed performance (e.g. Parker and Kulik, 1995). However, as far as objective performance measures are concerned, positive correlations are found as well. For instance, Keijsers *et al.* (1995) obtained an objective measure of ICU performance by calculating for each unit a standard mortality ratio—the ratio of actual versus predicted death rates adjusted for several patient characteristics such as diagnosis and severity of illness. Contrary to expectations, they found a small but significant positive correlation of objective ICU performance with emotional exhaustion (explained variance 2%) and no relationship with depersonalisation or personal accomplishment. It appeared that nurses felt exhausted who were employed in objectively and subjectively well-performing ICUs but who scored low on self-reported personal accomplishment. A possible explanation is that nurses in well-performing ICUs exert themselves more, and as a consequence feel more exhausted. An alternative explanation is that nurses in well-performing units have a higher standard of comparison and thus feel that they accomplish less. At any rate, it appears that—in contrast to the prevailing view—burnout is not necessarily linked to low levels of *actual* performance.

In summary, various correlates of burnout in health care have been identified. The most consistent and strong relationships – particularly with emotional exhaustion—are found with general job stressors such as workload, time pressure, role problems, and lack of social support. Relationships with specific job stressors pertaining to interactions with patients, as well as with personality factors, and with negative outcomes such as individual health, withdrawal from the organisation, and poor work performance are somewhat less strong. Strictly speaking, to date few causes or consequences of burnout have been identified, probably because the considerable stability of burnout across time—about 40–45% of the variance of burnout is explained by the level of burnout one year before (Schaufeli and Enzmann, 1998, pp. 96–97)—leaves little room for other causal factors.

PSYCHOLOGICAL EXPLANATIONS

Many different psychological explanations exist for burnout that emphasise the importance of individual, interpersonal, organisational, and societal factors respectively (for an overview see Schaufeli and Enzmann, 1998, pp. 100–142). This final section concentrates on two particular interpersonal approaches that are assumed to be of special importance for explaining burnout in health care because they emphasise the role of emotionally demanding relationships with patients.

Burnout as emotional overload

According to Maslach (1993), interpersonal demands resulting from the helping relationship are considered to be the root cause of burnout. She argues that patient contacts are emotionally charged by their very nature because health care professionals deal with troubled people who are in need. In order to deal with emotional demands and perform efficient and well, professionals may adopt techniques of detachment. When patients are treated in a more remote, objective way, it becomes easier to do one's job without suffering strong psychological discomfort. A functional way to do this is to develop an attitude of detached concern—the medical profession's ideal blending of compassion with emotional distance. A dysfunctional way is depersonalisation: a persistently callous, indifferent and cynical perception of patients. Ironically, the structure of the helping relationships in health care is such that it promotes this dysfunctional strategy. For instance, the focus is on the patients' problems rather than on their positive aspects and there is a lack of positive feedback from patients since they only return when things go wrong. As a result of depersonalisation, quality of care is likely to deteriorate because the major vehicle for the success—compassion with and concern for others—has been destroyed in an attempt to protect psychological integrity. Because success is increasingly lacking, the professional's sense of personal accomplishment erodes and feelings of inadequacy and self-doubt develop.

Based on the theoretical approach of Maslach, Leiter (1993) conducted a series of studies among health care workers in which he distinguished quantitative job demands (e.g., work overload, hassles), qualitative job demands (e.g., interpersonal conflict), and lack of resources (e.g., lack of social support, poor patient co-operation, lack of autonomy, and poor participation in decision making). As Figure 2.1 shows, demands were expected to be related with emotional exhaustion, whereas resources were expected to be related with depersonalisation and lack of personal accomplishment. Indeed, Leiter's results largely confirmed the hypothesised model. High job demands led to emotional exhaustion which then led to depersonalisation.

Contrary to the model, however, personal accomplishment seemed to develop rather independently from both emotional exhaustion and depersonalisation. Indeed, Leiter described it as developing in parallel with these two burnout dimensions, provided that resources were lacking of course. Recently, Lee and Ashforth (1996) concluded that the results of

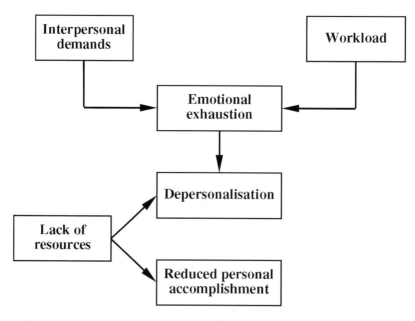

Figure 2.1:   Leiter's process model of burnout (after Leiter, 1993, p. 245)

their meta-analysis are largely consistent with Leiter's (1993) mixed sequential and parallel development model of burnout.

Burnout as lack of reciprocity

By definition, the professionals' relationship with patients is complementary, which is semantically well-illustrated by the terms "caregiver" and "recipient"; the former is supposed to give care, assistance, advice, support and so on, whereas the latter is supposed to receive them. Nevertheless, professionals look for some rewards in return for their efforts; for example, they expect their patients to show gratitude, to improve, or at least make a real effort to get well. Because, in practice, these expectations are seldom fulfilled it is likely that a lack of reciprocity develops over time: professionals feel that they continuously put much more into relationships with their patients than they receive in return. As Buunk and Schaufeli (1993) have pointed out, lack of reciprocity—an unbalanced helping relationship—drains the professionals' emotional resources and eventually leads to emotional exhaustion. This is typically dealt with by decreasing one's investments in the relationships with patients: that is, responding to patients in a depersonalised way instead of expressing genuine empathic concern. Accordingly, depersonalisation can be regarded as a way of restoring reciprocity by withdrawing psychologically from patients. However, this way of coping with an unbalanced interpersonal relationship is dysfunctional since it deteriorates the helping relationship, increases failures and thus fosters a sense of diminished personal accomplishment. Indeed, positive relationships were found between lack of reciprocity at the interpersonal level and all three dimensions of burnout among various health professionals such as student-nurses (Schaufeli et al., 1996), general hospital nurses (Schaufeli and Janczur, 1994) and general practitioners (Van Dierendonck et al., 1994).

Similar social exchange processes that are observed in interpersonal relationships govern the relationship of the professional with his or her organisation. Therefore, Schaufeli et al. (1996) have proposed a dual-level social exchange model (see Figure 2.2).

They argue that in addition to an unbalanced relationship at the interpersonal level, burnout is also caused by lack of reciprocity at the organisational level—that is, by a violation of the psychological contract. A psychological contract refers to the expectations held by employees about the nature of their exchange with the organisation. Expectations concern concrete issues such as workload, as well as less tangible matters such as esteem and dignity at work, and support from supervisors and colleagues. Thus, the psychological contract reflects the employees' subjective notion of reciprocity: they expect gains or outcomes from the

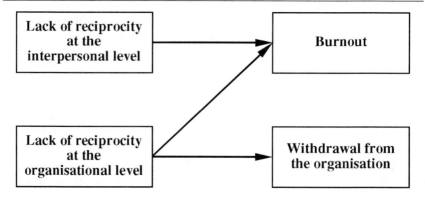

Figure 2.2:   The dual-level social exchange model of burnout (source: Schaufeli *et al.*, 1996, p. 228)

organisation that are proportional to their investments or inputs. When the psychological contract is violated because experience does not match expectancies, reciprocity is corroded. Schaufeli *et al.* (1996) argued that in addition to cognitive and behavioural withdrawal from the organisation (reduced organisational commitment, turnover and absenteeism), violation of the contract may also lead to burnout. The dual-level model was tested successfully in two samples of student-nurses (Schaufeli *et al.*, 1996). Moreover, recent studies among therapists from a forensic psychiatric clinic, and staff working with clients with learning difficulties, confirmed that burnout is related to perceptions of inequity at the organisational level (Van Dierendonck *et al.*, 1996) and that those perceptions can be altered, leading to less emotional exhaustion and less absenteeism (Van Dierendonck *et al.*, 1998).

It seems that a lack of reciprocity is a key concept for understanding burnout in health care. Instead of simply working too long and too hard with difficult recipients—as is assumed in most traditional approaches to burnout—it appears that the balance between investments and outcomes is crucial for its development. It looks like this mechanism is working in similar ways at the interpersonal level of care giver and patient, and at the organisational level of professional and organisation.

SUMMARY

To date, reliable estimates of the prevalence of burnout in health care do not exist, but it seems to be a serious problem given the huge attention it has drawn in past decades from researchers and practitioners. Burnout is related to job stress and depression but can nevertheless be distinguished from these conditions on conceptual as well as empirical grounds. Comparisons with other occupational fields revealed that typical burnout profiles exist in health care with physicians, for instance experiencing high levels of depersonalisation and nurses suffering from reduced personal accomplishment. On the empirical level, burnout—particularly emotional exhaustion—was found to be related with many other variables, including personality factors, job stressors, and individual and organisational outcomes. Theoretical approaches that emphasise the social nature of burnout by either taking into account the emotional overload resulting from patient contacts, or the disturbed balance between give and take, seem to offer a promising route for explaining burnout in health care settings and addressing it.

REFERENCES

Buunk, B.P. and Schaufeli, W.B. (1993). Burnout: A perspective from social comparison theory. In W.B. Schaufeli, C. Maslach and T. Marek (Eds), *Professional Burnout: Recent Developments in Theory and Research* (53–69). Washington, DC: Taylor & Francis.

Cordes, C.L. and Dougherty, T.W. (1993). A review and an integration of research on job burnout. *Academy of Management Review*, **18**, 621–656.

Corrigan, P.W., Holmes, E.P. and Luchins, D. (1995). Burnout and collegial support in state psychiatric hospital staff. *Journal of Clinical Psychology*, **51**, 703–710.

Firth, H. and Britton, P.G. (1989). "Burnout", absence and turnover amongst British nursing staff. *Journal of Occupational Psychology*, **62**, 55–59.

Garden, A.M. (1991). The purpose of burnout: A Jungian interpretation. *Journal of Social Behavior and Personality*, **6**, 73–93.

Glass, D.C. and McKnight, J.D. (1996). Perceived control, depressive symptomatology, and professional burnout: A review of the evidence. *Psychology and Health*, **11**, 23–48.

Keijsers, G.J., Schaufeli, W.B., Le Banc, P.M., Zwerts, C. and Reis-Miranda, D. (1995). Performance and burnout in intensive care units. *Work and Stress*, **9**, 513–527.

Landsbergis, P.A. (1988). Occupational stress among health care workers: A test of the job demands-control model. *Journal of Organizational Behavior*, **9**, 217–239.

Lee, R.T. and Ashforth, B.E. (1996). A meta-analytic examination of the correlates of the three dimensions of job burnout. *Journal of Applied Psychology*, **81**, 123–133.

Leiter, M.P. (1993). Burnout as a developmental process: consideration of models. In W.B. Schaufeli, C. Maslach and T. Marek (Eds) *Professional Burnout: Recent Developments in Theory and Research* (pp. 237–250). Washington, DC: Taylor & Francis.

Leiter, M.P. and Durup, M.J. (1996). Work, home, and in-between: A longitudinal study of spillover. *Journal of Applied Behavioral Science*, **32**, 29–47.

Mallett, K.L., Price, J.H., Jurs, S.G. and Slenker, S. (1991). Relationships among burnout, death anxiety, and social support in hospice and critical care nurses. *Psychological Reports*, **68**, 1347–1359.

Maslach, C. (1993). Burnout: a multidimensional perspective. In W.B. Schaufeli, C. Maslach and T. Marek (Eds) *Professional Burnout: Recent Developments in Theory and Research* (pp. 19–32). Washington, DC: Taylor & Francis.

Maslach, C. and Schaufeli, W.B. (1993). Historical and conceptual development of burnout. In W.B. Schaufeli, C. Maslach and T. Marek (Eds) *Professional Burnout: Recent Developments in Theory and Research* (pp. 1–16). Washington, DC: Taylor & Francis.

Maslach, C., Jackson, S.E. and Leiter, M. (1996). *Maslach Burnout Inventory. Manual* (3rd edn). Palo Alto, CA: Consulting Psychologists Press (1st edn, 1981; 2nd edn, 1996).

Parker, P.A. and Kulik, J.A. (1995). Burnout, self- and supervisor-rated job performance, and absenteeism among nurses. *Journal of Behavioral Medicine*, **18**, 581–599.

Pines, A.M. (1993). Burnout: an existential perspective. In W.B. Schaufeli, C. Maslach and T. Marek (Eds) *Professional Burnout: Recent Developments in Theory and Research* (pp. 33–51). Washington, DC: Taylor & Francis.

Schaufeli, W.B. and Janczur, B. (1994). Burnout among nurses. a Polish–Dutch comparison. *Journal of Cross-Cultural Psychology*, **25**, 95–113.

Schaufeli, W.B. and Enzmann, D. (1998) *The Burnout Companion to Study and Practice: A Critical Analysis*. London: Taylor & Francis.

Schaufeli, W.B. and Van Dierendonck, D. (1993). The construct validity of two burnout measures. *Journal of Organizational Behavior*, **14**, 631–647.

Schaufeli, W.B., Enzmann, D. and Girault, N. (1993). Measurement of burnout: a review. In W.B. Schaufeli, C. Maslach and T. Marek (Eds) *Professional Burnout: Recent Developments in Theory and Research* (pp. 199–215). Washington, DC: Taylor & Francis.

Schaufeli, W.B., Keijsers, G.J. and Reis-Miranda, D. (1995). Technology use, burnout, and performance in Intensive Care Units. In S.L. Sauter and L.R. Murphy (Eds) *Organizational Risk Factors for Job Stress* (pp. 259–271). Washington, DC: American Psychological Association.

Schaufeli, W.B., Van Dierendonck, D. and Van Gorp, K. (1996). Burnout and reciprocity: Towards a dual-level social exchange model. *Work and Stress*, **3**, 225–237.

Sixma, H.J., Bakker, A.B., Bosveld, W., Lobach, E., Groenewegen, P.P. and Schaufeli, W.B. (1998). *Dropping out as a consequence of burnout: a longitudinal study among Dutch general practitioners* (manuscript submitted for publication).

Van Dierendonck, D., Schaufeli, W.B. and Buunk, B.P. (1996). Inequality among human service professionals: measurement and relation to burnout. *Basic and Applied Social Psychology*, **18**, 429–451.

Van Dierendonck, D., Schaufeli, W.B. and Buunk, B.P. (1998). The evaluation of an individual burnout program. The role of inequity and social support. *Journal of Applied Psychology*, **83**, 392–407.

Van Dierendonck, D., Schaufeli, W.B. and Sixma, H.J. (1994). Burnout among general practitioners: a perspective from equity theory. *Journal of Social and Clinical Psychology*, **13**, 86–100.

3

INDIVIDUAL DIFFERENCES IN THE JOB STRESS PROCESS OF HEALTH CARE PROFESSIONALS

Paul E. Spector

Since their jobs deal with the health and well-being of others, the study of job stress is particularly appropriate for health care professionals. In recent years there has been increased interest in the role of personality in the job stress process. This represents a shift in emphasis away from purely environmental factors as an explanation for work stress. It recognises significant individual differences in perceptions of, and reactions to, environmental conditions normally considered to be job stressors. In particular, affective dispositions (e.g. trait anger and trait anxiety) and locus of control (the tendency to believe an individual does or does not control rewards in life) have been prominent as they represent important theoretical variables in the job stress process.

In this chapter current research and theorising about these personality variables will be summarised, with the focus on specific job conditions and experiences relevant to health care professionals. Although personality may play the same role in the job stress process regardless of whether the person is a physician or plumber, the incidents encountered

Stress in Health Professionals. Edited by Jenny Firth-Cozens and Roy L. Payne
© 1999 John Wiley & Sons Ltd

can be very different. The framework described in Payne's chapter (Chapter 4) will be used to organise this chapter; that is, it will look at job stressors, job stresses and the influence of personality on them.

MAJOR COMPONENTS OF THE JOB STRESS PROCESS

Job stressors

In general, health care jobs have been characterised as demanding, with a high degree of responsibility. Errors can have catastrophic effects on both the patient and the professional. A Dutch study compared health care workers with those in 18 other categories ranging from agriculture and construction to education and professional services (Houtman and Kompier, 1995). Health care workers were second of all categories to professional services occupations on the pace at which they worked. Within the various health care occupations, however, there can be considerable differences in job stressors.

The job of nurse has a high level of responsibility and workload, while at the same time having to deal with conflicting demands and often inadequate knowledge (Schaufeli *et al.*, 1995). In addition, nurses, as well as other health care workers, are exposed to both emotional and physical danger (McIntosh, 1995). Emotional danger comes from exposure to human pain and suffering, which can induce negative emotions, such as depression. Physical danger comes from exposure to infectious disease and toxic substances, as well as physical abuse from patients in emergency wards.

Although many job stressors are similar for most health care professionals, there are differences, especially when comparing occupations that differ in status and training. Menon *et al.*, (1996) collected data on three job stressors in samples of nurses and physicians. The nurses reported higher levels of situational constraints and workload than did physicians, but the physicians had higher levels of interpersonal conflict than did the nurses. These authors speculated that control differences were the likely reason for the discrepancy in results. Nurses who felt they had low control over their jobs were less able to reduce constraints and regulate their own workloads. Physicians, who had much more control over their work situation, were more likely to get into conflicts, perhaps over control issues, with colleagues and subordinates.

Even among nurses, there can be differences in job stressors depending upon the type of job one has. Parkes (1982) studied job stress among nurses who rotated between medical and surgical units of a hospital. She found that job stressors were higher in medical units, possibly due to longer patient stays and a higher patient mortality rate. Ogus (1995) noted differences in ability to handle stressors between general ward nurses, many of whom have relatively little experience, and more experienced and specialised intensive care nurses. The greater experience of the intensive care nurses gives them a greater repertoire of responses with which to cope with job stressors.

Job stress

Research on the job stress of health care professionals is somewhat conflicting. Some studies show relatively low levels of physical and psychological stress compared to other occupations (e.g. Houtman and Kompier, 1995), despite the fact that job stressors can be quite high. However, for at least some health-related occupations, job stress can be quite high. For example, Beaton et al. (1995) compared paramedics/firefighters to the more general population. The paramedics/firefighters were higher on anxiety and what are considered stress-related physical symptoms, such as gastro-intestinal symptoms and sleep disturbance. It seems likely that certain types of stressors contribute to certain types of stress. Some health care occupations might have high levels of stressors (e.g. workload), but the high workload does not necessarily lead to higher stress levels. Other health workers, such as the paramedics, may be frequently exposed to job stressors that are more conducive to producing ongoing work stresses.

Comparisons have been made among different health care professions. Nurses have been compared to higher status pharmacists and physicians. Wolfgang (1995) found that pharmacists reported less stress and higher job satisfaction than nurses. Menon et al. (1996) found that nurses reported more physical health symptoms than physicians, but the two groups did not differ in job satisfaction. Although it is not clear why these differences occurred, it is likely that they reflect the lower level of control by nurses than these other occupations that require greater training. There is, however, one addition factor to keep in mind. With many of these comparisons, gender is confounded with job. Lower level jobs, such as nurse, tend to be held by women, while higher level jobs, such as pharmacist or physician, are mainly held by men. For example, in Wolfgang's (1995) study, 97% of nurses were female and 73% of pharmacists were male. However, it seems unlikely that gender accounts for all of the results found. Differences between men and women on job stressors and job stress are typically small (e.g. Frone et al., 1995). Furthermore, gender does not seem to affect relations between job stressors and stress. For example, Barnett and Brennan (1997) found in a longitudinal study that there were no significant differences between men and women in the size of the relationships between job stressors and stress symptoms.

Even within the nursing profession, there are differences in job stress. Parkes (1982) found higher levels of psychological stress, such as depression, in medical as opposed to surgical units among nurses who were rotated through each. Ogus (1995) also found higher strain in medical units as compared to surgical. Burnout was higher in the medical units, especially the component of emotional exhaustion.

Personality and the job stress process

Affective dispositions
The term affective disposition refers to a family of personality traits that reflect an individual's tendency to experience specific emotional states across situations and time. Trait anxiety is the tendency to experience anxiety across situations. Individuals who are characterised as trait anxious are more likely to respond to situations with increased symptoms of anxiety. This is not to say that such individuals are necessarily in a chronic emotional state; rather they seem to be hyper-responsive to particular types of situation, and respond anxiously. Spielberger (1972) discussed how trait anxious people experience heightened anxiety in response to social stressors that threatened self-esteem, but not to physical stressors. This variable, therefore, is important for psychosocial job stressors (e.g. interpersonal conflict or role conflict) but not necessarily for physical job stressors (e.g. heat or overwork). Individuals who are high in trait anxiety are likely to avoid stressful jobs, and might be unlikely to seek the most stressful health care occupations. Studies have shown that high trait anxious individuals are more likely to be found in simpler, presumably less demanding jobs, than low trait anxious individuals (Spector et al., in press).

Trait anger is the tendency to experience anger across situations. As opposed to anxiety, much of the research on anger has focused on separating its experience from its expression (e.g. Spielberger et al., 1988). The experience of anger refers only to feelings of the emotion, while the expression refers to behaviours closely associated with the emotion, such as aggressive responses or yelling. In the stress domain, there is evidence that the way an individual deals with or expresses anger can have effects on stress (e.g., Greenglass, 1996; Julkunen, 1996). Individuals who are frequently angry and cannot deal with their anger constructively are more likely to develop cardiovascular disease.

Affective dispositions influence how people perceive the environment and emotional responses to those perceptions. Individuals who are high in trait anger or anxiety will be predisposed to interpret the environment as provoking or threatening. People who are low on this trait and are not easily roused to anger or anxiety, are less likely to see the environment in this way, and thus may interpret the same situations as being benign. Thus in this model affective dispositions serve as a cause of perceived job stressors, although they might serve a more complex and interactive role. A very low stress environment might be seen this way by almost everyone. The high anxious person will not likely become anxious in the absence of any demands at all, and might be just as calm as an individual who is low in trait anxiety. As job stressors begin to increase, the high anxious will respond immediately, with the low anxious not responding until perhaps a moderate level is achieved. Thus the high anxious person would be best suited to jobs with relatively low levels of job stressors, saving the highest stress jobs for the low anxious.

There have been many studies linking measures of affective dispositions to both perceived job stressors and job stress. Results with trait anxiety have consistently shown a link, although correlations with specific measures of job stressors and stress vary across studies in some cases. On the job stressor side, high trait anxiety has been associated with high levels of perceived interpersonal conflict, role ambiguity, role conflict, situational constraints and skill under-utilisation, and perceived low levels of autonomy (Chen and Spector, 1991; Fox and Spector, in press; Jex and Spector, 1996; Moyle, 1995; Sargent and Terry, 1994; Spector and O'Connell, 1994). These relations support the idea that high trait anxious people perceive more job stressors. However, one must be cautious in interpreting this to mean that the effect is only in perception. Spector *et al.* (in press) discuss considerable evidence suggesting that the high trait anxious might experience more objective job stressors than their low trait anxious counterparts. For example, a high trait anxious individual might perform poorly, and, as a consequence, receive constant pressure from a supervisor to improve.

Fewer studies have attempted to link trait anger to perceptions of job stressors. However, there is at least some evidence that a connection exists here as well, with the high anger individuals perceiving more job stressors. Fox and Spector (in press) have conducted one of the few studies showing such a link. They showed that trait anger was associated with perceptions of organisational constraints, but they did not report results with other job stressors.

On the job stress side, research again supports a role for affective dispositions. Evidence can be found showing that high trait anxiety is associated with higher absence from work, frustration, health symptoms, job dissatisfaction, poor well-being, and work-related anxiety (Chen and Spector, 1991; Jex and Spector, 1996; Moyle, 1995; Sargent and Terry, 1994; Spector and O'Connell, 1994). Relations with psychological stresses , such as job dissatisfaction tend to be larger than with other types of strains, such as absence. Fox and Spector (in press) found that high trait anxious individuals reported performing more counterproductive acts at work (e.g. sabotage and verbal aggression) than the low trait anxious. Such behaviours can be considered a form of coping, which can be emotionally helpful to the individual, at least in the short run, but detrimental to organisations.

Trait anger has also been linked to job stress, although again not many studies are available. Fox and Spector (in press) found in a sample of employees whose work involved computers that the high trait angry reported more frustration at work and less job satisfaction than low trait angry employees. Here again trait anger was linked to counterproductive work behaviour, such as arguing with others or sabotaging their work. Interestingly, where trait anxiety correlated more strongly with acts directed against the organisation than other people ($r = 0.40$ vs 0.20, respectively), trait anger correlated almost the same with both, and with larger correlations ($r = 0.57$ vs 0.50, respectively).

Locus of control

Locus of control refers to an individual's belief that he or she controls personally relevant outcomes in life. Individuals who are at one end of the continuum (internals) believe they are in control while their counterparts at the other end (externals) believe that luck or powerful others control outcomes in life. Although much of the early locus of control work was done with general scales, more recent research has been done to develop domain-specific scales. Most relevant to the job stress domain is the work locus of control scale (WLCS; Spector 1988, 1992), which assesses beliefs about control at work rather than life in general. Feelings of control in general, and locus of control in particular, are associated with low levels of psychological stress. People experience less negative emotion when they feel in control of their jobs and lives.

Locus of control is also hypothesised to influence perceptions of the environment. In general, situations that are seen as uncontrollable are perceived as more stressful both on and off the job (Averill, 1973; Thompson, 1981). Externals because of their tendency to believe they have little control, are more likely to perceive conditions or situations as being job stressors. Thus locus of control may influence perceptions of job stressors and also affect whether or not people will perceive job stressors. This perception of job stressors can lead to greater job stress, particularly to emotions such as anger or anxiety. In addition, locus of control can influence people's behavioural reactions when they perceive job stressors. Individuals who believe they have little control are more likely to resort to counterproductive behaviour, such as aggression or sabotage, in response to job stressors that induce anger (e.g. Allen and Greenberger,

1980). Here again, externals will be more likely to perceive low control in situations, which will lead to a greater likelihood of their getting angry and committing counterproductive acts as a result.

There is research support for a link between locus of control and both job stressors and job stress. Locus of control correlates with employee reports of the job stressors of lack of control, organisational constraints, role ambiguity, and role conflict (Fox and Spector, in press; Sargent and Terry, 1994; Spector, 1988; Spector and O'Connell, 1994), with externals reporting higher levels of all of these job stressors. Externals also tend to report higher levels of job stress, including counterproductive behaviour, frustration, job dissatisfaction, and work anxiety (Fox and Spector, in press; Moyle, 1995; Sargent and Terry, 1994; Spector, 1988; Spector and O'Connell, 1994). Furthermore, Perlow and Latham (1993) found that locus of control predicted which employees would be caught abusing residents of a facility for the developmentally disabled. Storms and Spector (1987) found support for the moderating effects of locus of control on relations between work frustration and counterproductive behaviour, among mental health employees. Frustrated externals, but not internals, were likely to respond counterproductively at work. In both of these studies, the employees were responsible for the care of others in either in-patient or out-patient settings.

CONCLUSIONS

Many health care occupations involve high workloads with demands for few errors. At the same time there are both emotional and physical dangers. The combination of both physical and psychosocial stressors can be perceived as quite stressful, especially for professionals with little control, such as nurses. As demonstrated, people vary in their tendencies to perceive job stressors and to experience job stress. Trait affectivity and locus of control have been shown to relate to both variables, but there are certainly other personality variables that are also important.

There are two implications of the findings discussed here. First, it might prove useful to use personality tests for the selection of health care workers for jobs that are unusually stressful, such as emergency room nurse or paramedic. For some jobs, individuals must be quite stress resistant to be able to perform well, particularly over a long period of time. Second, organisations should be flexible in dealing with problems of job stress, especially among those individuals who are most prone to be affected. There are likely to be some individuals in every organisation who are relatively external and high in trait anxiety and other affective traits. Since personality characteristics such as affective dispositions and locus of control are relatively stable and not easily modified, organisations might look to interventions that might be helpful. For example, offering enhanced control, or helping individuals to recognise the control they have, can be effective in reducing perceived stressors and in encouraging more productive means of coping. Chapters 14, 15 and 16 of this volume give detailed examples of interventions to cope with work stress which are also sensitive to the role of personality in the process. Since individual differences are important influences on perceptions of job stressors and experience of job stress, interventions should allow for such differences to enhance effectively the health and well-being of health care professionals.

REFERENCES

Allen, V.L. and Greenberger, D.B. (1980). Destruction and perceived control. In A. Baum and J.E. Singer (Eds) *Applications of Personal Control*, (Vol. 2) (pp. 85–109). Hillsdale, NJ: Lawrence Erlbaum.

Averill, J. (1973). Personal control over aversive stimuli and its relationship to stress. *Psychological Bulletin*, **80**, 286–303.

Barnett, R.C. and Brennan, R.T. (1997). Change in job conditions, change in psychological distress, and gender: a longitudinal study of dual-earner couples. *Journal of Organizational Behavior*, **18**, 253–274.

Beaton, R., Murphy, S., Pike, K. and Jarrett, M. (1995). Stress-symptom factors in firefighters and paramedics. In S.L. Sauter and L.R. Murphy (Eds) *Organizational Risk Factors for Job Stress* (pp. 227–245). Washington, DC: American Psychological Association.

Chen, P.Y. and Spector, P.E. (1991). Negative affectivity as the underlying cause of correlations between stressors and strains. *Journal of Applied Psychology*, **76**, 398–407.

Fox, S. and Spector, P.E. (in press). A model of work frustration-aggression. *Journal of Organizational Behavior*.

Frone, M.R., Russell, M. and Cooper, M.L. (1995). Job stressors, job involvement and employee health: a test of identity theory. *Journal of Occupational and Organizational Psychology*, **68**, 1–11.

Greenglass, E.R. (1996). Anger suppression, cynical distrust, and hostility: implications for coronary heart disease. In C.D. Spielberger, I.G. Sarason, J.M.T. Brebner, E. Greenglass, P. Laungani and A.M. O'Roark (Eds) *Stress and Emotion: Anxiety, Anger, and Curiosity*, Vol. 16 (pp. 205–225). Washington, DC: Taylor & Francis.

Hackett, R.D. and Bycio, P. (1996). An evaluation of employee absenteeism as a coping mechanism among hospital nurses. *Journal of Occupational and Organizational Psychology*, **69**, 327–338.

Houtman, I.L.D. and Kompier, M.A.J. (1995). Risk factors and occupational risk groups for work stress in the Netherlands. In S.L. Sauter and L.R. Murphy (Eds) *Organizational Risk Factors for Job Stress* (pp. 209–225). Washington, DC: American Psychological Association.

Jex, S.M. and Spector, P.E. (1996). The impact of negative affectivity on stressor—strain relations: A replication and extension. *Work and Stress*, **10**, 36–45.

Julkunen, J. (1996). Suppressing your anger: good manners, bad health? In C.D. Spielberger, I.G. Sarason, J.M.T. Brebner, E. Greenglass, P. Laungani and A.M. O'Roark (Eds) *Stress and Emotion: Anxiety, Anger, and Curiosity*, Vol. 16 (pp. 227–240). Washington, DC: Taylor & Francis.

Lazarus, R.S. and Folkman, S. (1984). *Stress, Appraisal and Coping*. New York: Springer.

McIntosh, N.J. (1995). Exhilarating work: an antidote for dangerous work? In S.L. Sauter and L.R. Murphy (Eds) *Organizational Risk Factors for Job Stress* (pp. 303–316). Washington, DC: American Psychological Association.

Menon, S., Narayanan, L. and Spector, P.E. (1996). Time urgency and its relation to occupational stressors and health outcomes for health care professionals In C.D. Spielberger, I.G. Sarason, J.M.T. Brebner, E. Greenglass, P. Laungani and A.M. O'Roark (Eds) *Stress and Emotion: Anxiety, Anger, and Curiosity*, Vol. 16 (pp. 127–142). Washington, DC: Taylor & Francis.

Moyle, P. (1995). The role of negative affectivity in the stress process: tests of alternative models. *Journal of Organizational Behavior*, **16**, 647–668.

O'Leary, A. (1990). Stress, emotion, and human immune function. *Psychological Bulletin*, **108**, 363–382.

Ogus, E.D. (1995). Burnout and coping strategies: a comparative study of ward nurses In R. Crandall and P.L. Perrewé (Eds) *Occupational Stress: A Handbook* (pp. 249–261). Washington, DC: Taylor & Francis.

Parkes, K.R. (1982). Occupational stress among student nurses: a natural experiment. *Journal of Applied Psychology*, **67**, 784–796.

Perlow, R. and Latham, L.L. (1993). Relationship of client abuse with locus of control and gender: A longitudinal study. *Journal of Applied Psychology*, **78**, 831–834.

Sargent, L. and Terry, D.J. (1994). The effects of work control and job demands on employee adjustment and work performance. Paper presented at the Annual Convention of the Academy of Management, Dallas, TX (August).

Schaufeli, W.B., Keijsers, G.J. and Miranda, D.R. (1995). Burnout, technology use, and ICU performance In S.L. Sauter and L.R. Murphy (Eds) *Organizational Risk Factors for Job Stress* (pp. 259–271). Washington, DC: American Psychological Association.

Spector, P.E. (1988). Development of the work locus of control scale. *Journal of Occupational Psychology*, **61**, 335–340.

Spector, P.E. (1992). A consideration of the validity and meaning of self-report measures of job conditions. In C.L. Cooper and I.T. Robertson (Eds) *International Review of Industrial and Organizational Psychology: 1992* (pp. 123–151). Chichester: Wiley.

Spector, P.E. and O'Connell, B.J. (1994). The contribution of individual dispositions to the subsequent perceptions of job stressors and job strains. *Journal of Occupational and Organizational Psychology*, **67**, 1–11.

Spector, P.E., Zapf, D., Chen, P.Y. and Frese, M. (in press). Why negative affectivity should not be controlled in job stress research: don't throw out the baby with the bath water. *Journal of Organizational Behavior*.

Spielberger, C.D. (1972). Anxiety as an emotional state. In C.D. Spielberger (Ed.) *Anxiety: Current trends in theory and research*, Vol. 1 (pp. 23–49). New York: Academic Press.

Spielberger, C.D., Krasner, S.S. and Solomon, E.P. (1988). The experience, expression and control of anger. In M.P. Janisse (Ed.) *Health psychology: Individual differences and stress* (pp. 89–108). New York: Springer.

Storms, P.L. and Spector, P.E. (1987). Relationships of organizational frustration with reported behavioral reactions: the moderating effect of perceived control. *Journal of Occupational Psychology*, **60**, 227–234.

Thompson, S.C. (1981). Will it hurt less if I can control it? A complex answer to a simple question. *Psychological Bulletin*, **90**, 89–101.

Wolfgang, A.P. (1995). Job stress, coping, and dissatisfaction in the health professions: a comparison of nurses and pharmacists In R. Crandall and P.L. Perrewé (Eds) *Occupational Stress: A Handbook* (pp. 193–204). Washington, DC: Taylor & Francis.

4

PSYCHOLOGICAL AND PHYSIOLOGICAL ASPECTS OF STRESS

Joe Herbert

STRESS: WHAT IS IT?

There is a danger that the use of the term "stress" will become so general and indefinite that it will cease to have any scientific value. This would be a pity, for stress can be defined, provided that this is done rigorously. We start with the idea of physiological homeostasis, originally proposed with such clarity by Claude Bernard. There are three essential components in homeostasis: the first is the means to detect external or internal agents that threaten to change some essential parameter (say, blood glucose); the second is the means to measure this parameter, and detect whether it falls within certain limits (these may themselves change in different circumstances); finally, there must be mechanisms to correct the incipient disturbance or to avoid its occurrence.

Consistent with its use in this book, a stressor is the general name given to any agent that tends to threaten homeostasis; stress is the effect this has on psychological and physiological systems; response to stress refers to the measures by which the individual copes with stress (sometimes called "strain"). "Stress", as it is often used, includes several components. Stress is a generic, not a specific, term. The essence of adaptation to, or coping with, stress is that there are (neural) mechanisms that detect and classify

Stress in Health Professionals. Edited by Jenny Firth-Cozens and Roy L. Payne
© 1999 John Wiley & Sons Ltd

the stress. So the detection of stress, and the response to it, is a differentiated one and the term "stress" includes a wide variety of conditions, all characterised by states of demand. No matter what the stress, there is a triad of responses to it, made up of behavioural, physiological and endocrine components. As we will see, there are well-characterised neural systems that detect and respond to the different categories of stresses.

Though physiological stresses (demands) are important, there are others, equally important. Besides the danger of predation (i.e. stress derived from other species), there are the most complex external stresses: social stress. Social groups act both as an aid to adaptation (that is, the group acts as a resource for the individual) but also as a source of stress. Con-specifics, including man, compete for access to resources that are necessarily scarce; for example, food, water, shelter and mates. This implies that there is a kind of social homeostasis; that is, there are mechanisms that detect and regulate this source of stress, and confer the means for adapting to it. There must, therefore, be neural and physiological mechanisms that not only detect and assess these complex stressors but also enable the individual to cope or adapt to them. A major concern of this chapter is to summarise how much we know of these mechanisms, and how effective they are.

Time is an important feature of stress. Although some stresses may be short-lived (blood-loss, for example, or being chased by an adversary), social stress may endure for years. Not only is the effect of time itself important—that is, the effect the stress has on the individual may be time- as well as stress-dependent—but the passage of time allows modulations to the way the stress is perceived, enables resources to deal with it to be recruited, and psychophysiological mechanisms modified. That is, there is reciprocal feedback between the stress, the response to it, and the "cost" (pathological reactions). This "transactional" view of stress as an evolving process is an influential one, and is an important component of the way that stress can lead to ill-health.

HORMONES

Changes in the level of hormones have long been known to accompany, and be part of, the response to stress. What is less obvious, in many cases, is whether these changes have functional importance.

Catecholamines

The adrenal gland is a major source for these stress-related events. The classical studies of Cannon established a role for the autonomic nervous system in "flight or fight" reactions; this includes secretion of catecholamine hormones (adrenaline and noradrenaline) from the adrenal medulla. The catecholamine hormones are inextricably linked with the cardiovascular system, on which they have potent actions, though coincident activation of the autonomic system (which also uses catecholamines as transmitters—i.e. local hormones) will also alter heart rate and blood pressure, etc. There has been some debate over the relative secretion of the two principal catecholamine hormones from the adrenal medulla—adrenaline and noradrenaline; proposals that predictable ratios accompanied specific emotional states have not been well supported by subsequent experimental or clinical findings. Whilst it is generally believed that catecholamine hormones are liberated in response to an acute stress (particularly those requiring much effort), there is evidence for more persistent elevation in subjects with chronic conditions, such as post-traumatic stress disorder (PTSD) (Southwick *et al.*, 1997; Yehuda *et al.*, 1998) or even post-operatively (Roth-Isigkeit *et al.*, 1998). Furthermore, those with chronic antecedent stress may show exaggerated rises in catecholamines (Pike *et al.*, 1997). However, chronic parental stress increased blood cortisol, but not catecholamines (Luecken *et al.*, 1997), whereas more acute marital conflict increased noradrenaline (but not adrenaline) (Kiecolt-Glaser *et al.*, 1997). Personality variables may affect catecholamine responses: for example, noradrenaline levels during harassment by a stooge were greater in men scoring highly on a "hostility" scale than those with lower scores (Suarez *et al.*, 1998). Current mental state may also influence catecholamine responses: for example, sub-clinical depressed mood enhanced noradrenaline responses to an acute stress (recalling anger) (Light *et al.*, 1998). Changes in peripheral catecholamines have limited roles in brain function, since the blood–brain barrier is highly impermeable to these hormones.

Cortisol

The classical studies of Selye (1956) firmly established increased secretion of glucocortocoids (principally cortisol in humans, corticosterone in rats) as an intrinsic feature of the response to stress. Nearly all mammals, including man, live in social groups. There is little doubt that an animal's position in the social hierarchy can be highly stressful. In monkey groups, the majority of aggressive interactions are directed towards more subordinate animals. This, and the threat of being attacked, seems to represent a potent form of chronic or persistent stress. This state is reflected by both behavioural and endocrine markers. A subordinate monkey shows high levels of vigilance, constantly monitoring the actions of more dominant animals (particularly those of the same sex) (Eberhart *et al.*, 1980, 1985) (Figure 4.1). There are equally marked disturbances in the diurnal rhythms of cortisol, with elevated levels throughout the day, most prominently in the evening (when cortisol is usually at its minimum) (Martensz et al., 1987) (Figure 4.1). Subordinate vervet monkeys show stress-typical lesions such as gastric ulcers; there may also be increased neuronal death rate in corticoid-sensitive areas of the brain such as the hippocampus (Sapolsky, 1986). Mortality rates are much higher in subordinate monkeys than in more dominant ones (Uno et al., 1989). In humans, as in experimental animals, it is uncontrollable or unpredictable stress that is particularly liable to increase blood cortisol (e.g. Peters et al., 1998). Persistently elevated cortisol may also impair mental health. The glucocorticoid receptors in the brain are only fully saturated (i.e. activated) by stress-increased levels of cortisol. High levels of glucocorticoids, whether therapeutic or pathological, are known to induce severe mood changes. Fifty per cent or more of those with Cushing's disease become depressed, and up to 75% of those on exogenous steroids for prolonged periods may develop mood disturbances (Kelly et al., 1983; Lewis and Smith, 1983; Wolkowitz, 1994).

Sex hormones

It is not often realised that reduced levels of gonadal hormones, particularly testosterone in men, are a sensitive and frequent correlate of stress. Studies on primate groups (as well as on other species) have shown that the state of subordination has profound effects on both sexual behaviour and on fertility. For example, the most subordinate males in a group of monkeys have lower testosterone levels than more dominant males, and also show very low levels of sexual activity (Yodyingyuad et al., 1982). Comparable findings have been described in men; the effects of persistent social stress on sexuality are both pervasive and profound (Herbert, 1996)

Other hormones

The focus on the three categories discussed above should not cloud the fact that the response to stress involves a wide range of hormones. Mason (1972) pointed out the variety and richness of the pattern of endocrine activation following stress, and suggested that this might differ according to the stressor.

THE ROLE OF THE BRAIN

The components needed to detect and react to stress, at their simplest, are: a detector to signal deviations from the acceptable range (e.g. levels

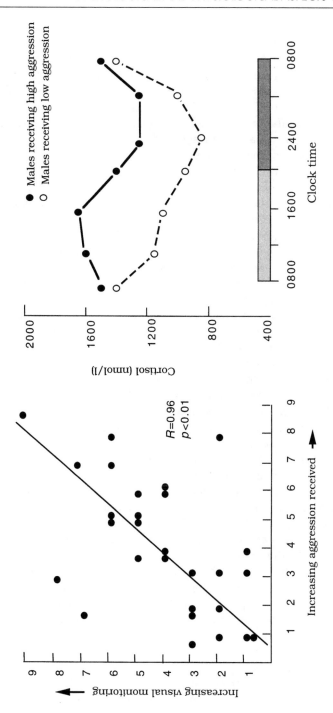

Figure 4.1: *Left:* the relation between a visual behaviour ('monitoring') and aggression in a group of monkeys; *right:* differences in the daily pattern of cortisol in monkeys receiving either high (i.e. subordinate) or low (i.e. dominant) amounts of aggression from other group members

of serum sodium) and an effector which can mount the appropriate set of responses. Following this analogy, we see that changes in sodium are detected by specific neurons in the hypothalamus ("osmo-receptors") located, it seems, in a restricted area of the anterior third ventricle. It is important to note that these neurons seem to be specific to this stimulus; other states (e.g. low blood glucose) are detected by other neurons (in this case, in the mid hypothalamus). The hypothalamus, then, contains series of neurons that signal changes in selected parameters of the internal environment and also organises a co-ordinated response to them. Hypothalamic lesions disturb the normal ability to respond to a physiological stress by appropriate behaviour, endocrine reactions and autonomic activation. There is little doubt that similar (but not identical) hypothalamic mechanisms are involved in responses to social stress.

There are a number of different methods by which to study the role of different parts of the nervous system in stress. The classical approach is to lesion a restricted area, and then determine how this alters some chosen dependent parameter of the response to a given stressor. This technique assumes that the "missing function" can be ascribed to the damaged area; it also depends upon the accuracy of the lesion and a consideration of what is destroyed (e.g. nerve cells only, or cells and intercurrent fibres?). Local alteration of function by electrical or chemical (e.g. pharmacological) methods has been less used, but can also be very informative though there are problems about localisation of the stimulus and its specificity. Alteration of genes, or gene products (e.g. peptide content) can reflect the way that the brain reacts to stress, and, in some cases, can have direct functional implications (e.g. can indicate whether a given neurotransmitter is part of the response to stress).

The expression (activation) of a class of genes called immediate-early genes (IEG) can be used as an indicator of neuronal activity, for example *c-fos*. This allows us to map the pattern of neural activity in experimental animals exposed to social stress (Figure 4.2). These studies allow two principal conclusions: they show that there is a distributed, but localised, pattern of neuronal activation in the brains of rats exposed to social stress. They also show that this pattern is modified during repeated exposure; that is, there is evidence of adaptation at the level of the neuron to social stress. The important point here is that not only does this happen, but it is uneven: that is, some groups of neurons show more rapid and more complete adaptation than others. This suggests that adaptation, at the neural level, is complex and that the overall process could vary according to circumstances. The major problem with the IEG technique is that, although we know that these genes act as transcriptional regulators (i.e. they regulate the activity of other, downstream genes) we have little idea of the identity of these genes in the context of the stress response.

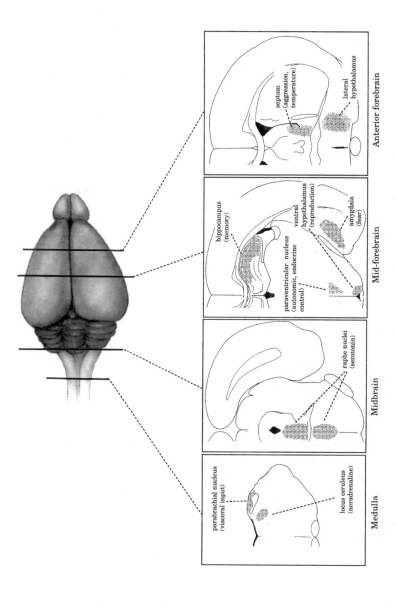

Figure 4.2: Diagrammatic representation of increased gene expression (*c-fos*) in the brains of rats following social stress. A series of cross-sections through the brain is shown, each one containing a specific area concerned with stress responses

Hypothalamus

The exact pattern of activation in the hypothalamus depends crucially upon the nature of the stress. For example, water deprivation (hypovolaemia) results in activity in a region lying around the anterior part of the third ventricle (so called AV3V), whereas lowered blood glucose activates areas in the medial hypothalamus. Social stress (as well as other categories) stimulates the paraventricular nucleus (PVN), a site now known to be important for both autonomic and endocrine responses. The neurons of the PVN express a large number of peptides, but two have been particularly implicated in stress. Corticotropin-releasing factor (CRF), a 41 amino-acid peptide, is expressed in part of the PVN (Figure 4.3). CRF has potent effects on behaviour (for example, it is anxiogenic and it increases aggression), on ACTH secretion from the anterior pituitary (and hence cortisol levels), and on autonomic activity (Berridge and Dunn, 1989; Cole *et al.*, 1990; Monnikes *et al.*, 1992; Thatcher-Britton *et al.*, 1986; Elkabir *et al.*, 1990). Expression of CRF tends to decrease after multiple stressors; however, arginine-vasopressin (AVP), another peptide, behaves differently. AVP has similar actions to CRF, but also synergises with CRF to increase the latter's potency; and expression of AVP tends to increase during persistent stress (Gillies *et al.*, 1982; Elkabir *et al.*, 1990; De Goeij *et al.*, 1991; Ma and Lightman, 1998). These results show the flexible nature of the neurochemical response in the brain to stress, and emphasise the role of peptides, molecules that exist in great profusion as neuromodulators and seem to be able to activate relatively specific patterns of adaptive responses (Herbert, 1993).

Pro-opiomelanocortin (POMC) is another peptide that seems to be closely involved in stress. This large peptide, the precursor for daughter peptides such as β-endorphin, ACTH (adrenocorticotropin hormone) and MSH (melanocyte-stimulating hormone) is found in another hypothalamic area, the arcuate nucleus (Figure 4.3). CRF may activate its expression (as it does in the pituitary); and POMC peptides have been implicated in the reproductive and ingestive effects of stress (Herbert, 1996). For example, β-endorphin infusions into the hypothalamus inhibit sexual behaviour in male rats (Hughes *et al.*, 1987). Other, simpler, physiological stress reactions are also dependent on peptides: for example, hypovolaemic-induced drinking is mediated by hypothalamic angiotensin (an octapeptide) (Fitzsimons, 1998). The general conclusion is that the hypothalamus is concerned with the organisation of co-ordinated responses to stress, and that this depends, at least in part, to selective activation of peptides, molecules that can carry a great deal of information.

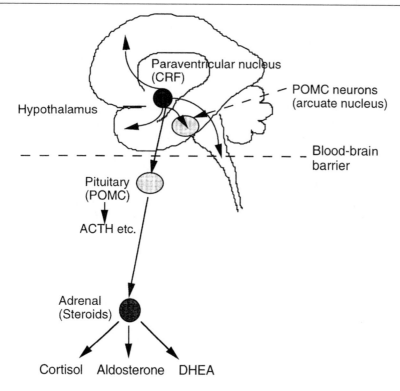

Figure 4.3: Diagrammatic representation of the interaction between the brain and the endocrine system. The brain contains groups of neurons (e.g. the paraventricular nucleus) that express peptides. These peptides have multiple but associated roles in the response to stress. In this example, the peptide CRF is shown acting on a variety of target organs, including sites in the brain but also on the pituitary gland, hence controlling the secretion of steroids from the adrenal. The blood–brain barrier is impermeable to peptides, but permeable to steroids

The amygdala

The amygdala receives extensive sensory input from the neocortex (Figure 4.4). The cortical association area for visual, auditory, tactile and gustatory information all project to the amygdala through the temporal neocortex. The amygdala also receives direct input from the olfactory bulbs and projections from polysensory convergence areas in frontal and temporal neocortex, as well an inputs from the sensory thalamus (Campeau and Davis, 1995). Projections from the amygdala pass to other parts of the limbic system, as well as the brainstem autonomic centres; there are also reciprocal pathways back to the cortex (Krettek and Price, 1976; Price et al., 1987) (Figure 4.4). The amygdaloid complex is involved in processes

determining the way in which the individual's brain perceives and inter-
prets a given stimulus or situation. Its central function is to associate a
sensory stimulus with an emotional response. A large body of experimental work shows that the amygdala is also concerned with the generation
of fear, including conditioned fear (that is, learning that previously neutral events may signal aversive events) (Maren and Fanselow, 1996; Kagan and Schulkin, 1995). Since the response to stress involves recognition
that external events are threatening, it is clear that the amygdala plays an
important role.

Damage to different nuclei of the amygdala can reduce stress responses, particularly those to conditioned (learned) stress. These include
cardiovascular activation (Roozendaal *et al.*, 1990), endocrine responses
(Roozendaal *et al.*, 1996) as well as behavioural ones (LeDoux, 1994). *C-fos*
expression in the amygdala (i.e. neural activation) is also increased by
either acute stress (e.g. footshocks; either unconditioned or conditioned)

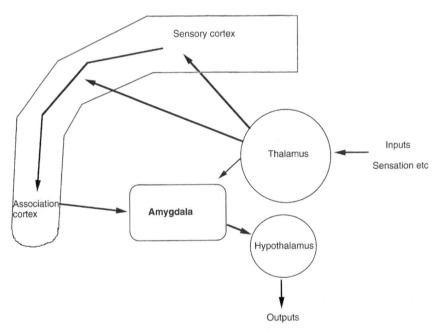

Figure 4.4: The relation of the amygdala to the rest of the brain (simplified).
Stress-related information flows into the brain through the thalamus, and hence to
the primary cortex. After processing (in the association cortex) information passes
to the amygdala, and then to the hypothalamus, which organises the requisite co-
ordinated (adaptive) outputs. Not shown are reciprocal projections from amygdala to cortex

or persistent social stress (e.g. aggression) (Campeau *et al.*, 1991; Martinez *et al.*, 1998). In man, although there is parallel evidence that the amygdala is concerned with fear (e.g. Adolphs *et al.*, 1995) there are no adequate studies of its role in the appreciation, analysis and response to persistent social stress. Extrapolating from the experimental findings suggests that the amygdala in man may have a critical role in the emotional response to stress, and the mechanisms whereby initially neutral stimuli acquire stress-associated qualities. However, the precise neural events that are responsible for these roles remain unknown.

Hippocampus

The focus has been on the response of the hippocampus to stress, rather than its role in the neural adaptation to it. The hippocampus seems curiously sensitive to a variety of damaging agents. There are also high densities of corticoid receptors on its neurons, and this may account for at least some of its response to stress. Prolonged exposure to high levels of circulating corticosterone in rats increased the age-related rate at which hippocampal pyramidal neurons are lost (Sapolsky,1996), and induced atrophy of apical dendrites (Magarinos and McEwen, 1995). Glucocorticoids have also been shown to potentiate neurodegeneration induced by anoxia, glutamate analogues such as kainic acid or cholinergic agents. In man, Cushing's syndrome, major depression and PTSD have all been associated with reduced hippocampal volumes (Gurvits *et al.*, 1996; Sheline *et al.*, 1996; Gebarski *et al.*, 1996). The functional implications of these findings are still uncertain. The hippocampus has been associated with spatial memory in rats, but with episodic memory in man. There is evidence that stress, or elevated corticoids, can impair cognitive function in humans (Porter and Landfield, 1998). It is becoming apparent that hippocampal damage may underlie some of the longer-term adverse neurological sequelae to stress.

Frontal cortex

The frontal cortex is essential for social learning, anticipation of the consequences of behaviour and response selection. Damage to the dorsolateral cortex in man impairs social judgement, and may have pervasive effects on cognition. The orbital part of the frontal lobe are well known to be concerned with emotional responses. Together, the frontal lobes are responsible for some of the most sophisticated functions of the brain and, as such, must play a crucial role in the appreciation, estimation and analysis of social stress. However, it must be said that much of the evidence (in man at least) on frontal lobe function is on more intellectual and cognitive functions, rather than its presumed role in complex social analysis. The frontal neocortex is intimately connected with both the amygdala and the hypothalamus and is therefore in a position to influence these other brain centres implicated in stress. The orbitofrontal cortex receives information from both external sensory sources and from the lower centres which regulate stress responses, and it projects back onto these lower centres. Humans with lesions in the orbitofrontal cortex react impulsively, without planning or taking into account the consequences of their behaviour. They experience brief outbursts of anger in response to demands during which they may take impulsive action and, after committing an aggressive act, are usually indifferent to the consequences (Luria, 1980). Thus, this region is implicated in the process that decides the time, place and strategy of response appropriate to demands from the environment. It seems likely that the frontal cortex plays a major part in the neural processing of emotional responses to stress (Davidson, 1992) and the way that social interactions are used to determine interpersonal relationships. This has obvious implications in the way that people react to, or deal with, social stress.

NEUROCHEMICAL RESPONSES TO STRESS

Dividing the brain into regions such as the hypothalamus, amygdala, frontal cortex and so on implies a view of the way that the brain is constructed and that definable functions can be ascribed to such anatomically defined regions. But the brain can also be viewed as a set of chemically defined systems, some of which are not congruent with the more traditional views of brain structure.

The monoamines (e.g. serotonin, noradrenaline, dopamine) are a set of such systems that have several features in common (Figure 4.5 and 4.6). All derive from small (but distinct) sets of neurons in the brainstem. All are distributed widely (but not uniformly) to the rest of the brain; in some cases (e.g. DA and NA) there are relatively distinct areas of apparent influence; in others (e.g. serotonin, NA) such distinctions are more subtle. Stress activates all three systems. NA responds to acute stress, but seems to accommodate rapidly (Martinez et al., 1998). Serotonin (5HT) shows more persistent activation. The release of DA in the frontal cortex is one of the more consistent results of exposing animals to stress (interestingly, release in other areas receiving DA—e.g. the striatum—may be less impressive). It seems evident that stress, by activating these chemically distinct, but related, neurochemical systems, results in widespread changes in the function of the brain. The majority of studies focus on one or other of monoaminergic systems. However, the true role of monoamines may

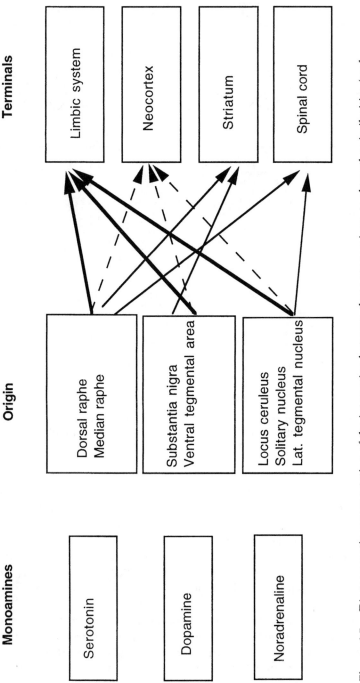

Figure 4.5: Diagrammatic representation of the interaction between three monamines, to show the similarities (and differences) between them

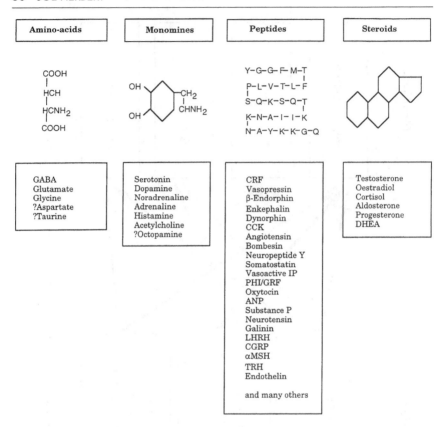

Figure 4.6: Chemical coding in the brain. Examples of the differences in structure of four classes of neurochemicals known to be concerned with information transfer in the brain

be a product of the relative activity of the several monoaminergic systems, but this question has hardly been addressed. Although the precise significance of these regulatory systems is not understood, despite decades of intense research, their implication in some of the pathological sequelae of social stress (e.g. major depression) indicates their potential importance. Other aminergic systems (e.g. acetylcholine) have many comparable features and may also belong to these systems in a functional sense.

Peptides are a second, biochemically distinct, class of neurochemical mediators (Figure 4.6) (Herbert, 1993). They are also found throughout the brain, though their distribution varies considerably. In contrast to monoamines, they often have rather specific roles to play. The huge number of peptides may represent a chemically coded "language" by which the limbic system operates a set of adaptive and regulatory instructions. The multiplicity of controls needed for each dependent function (for example, food intake, water balance, etc.) is reflected in the equally large number of neuropeptides devoted to such functions. For example, food intake is powerfully regulated by several peptides, including CRF, leptins, NPY, cholecystokinin, opioids, orexins. This reflects the multiple regulation (both short and longer term) of this essential function. Peptides also serve to co-ordinate responses to a given demand: for example, angiotensin II in the brain increases thirst, raises blood pressure, and stimulates the secretion of vasopressin (Fitzsimons, 1998): together, these represent a highly effective adaptive response to water deprivation or hypovolaemia. CRF and vasopressin (AVP) increase "anxiety"-like behaviour, as well as stimulating the autonomic system and adrenal hormones: all are part of the co-ordinated response to social (and other) stress (Herbert, 1993). Infusions of different peptides (e.g. angiotensin II, CRF, NPY, etc.) into the brain induce peptide-specific patterns of *c-fos* expression, indicating that peptides activate distributed, but related, groups of neurons (Herbert *et al.*, 1992; Andreae and Herbert, 1993; Arnold *et al.*, 1992). CRF in the CSF levels have been found to be raised in depressive illness (Nemeroff *et al.*, 1984), though whether CRF contributes to the symptoms of this condition remains uncertain. The powerful and restricted actions of peptides make them prime candidates for encoding specific components of the neural response to stress, both adaptive and pathological. But there is much more to be learned of their precise roles.

The steroids are the third component of this chemically specified system (Figure 4.6). They have been discussed in some detail above; here it is only necessary to note that they enter the brain from the circulation (though there is increasing evidence that the brain can itself make steroids) and thus interact, at receptor level, with the amines and peptides.

Together, these three systems seem to determine the nature and efficacy of the individual's response to stress.

STRESS AND DEPRESSION

It is now well-established that psychosocial adversity (stress) is a powerful contributing factor to major depressive disorder (MDD). Both retrospective and prospective studies show that persistent adversity ("difficulties"), often followed by a more dramatic "precipitating" event (a "life event") is likely to be followed by the appearance of depressive illness in some—but certainly not all—individuals experiencing these social conditions (Brown and Harris, 1989; Paykel and Cooper, 1992). Disturbances in cortisol have long been known to be associated with MDD; recently, lowered DHEA (dehydroepiandrosterone), a second adrenal steroid, has been found in cases of depression in both adolescents and adults (Goodyer *et al.*, 1996; Michael *et al.*, unpublished data). DHEA can counteract the neural actions of cortisol, and is neuroprotective (Kimonides *et al.*, 1998). It remains to be seen whether changes in either cortisol, DHEA or both are induced by social stress, and contribute to the later development of MDD. Of course, MDD is not the only stress-associated illness and steroids are not the only systems sensitive to stress (see above); our understanding of the role of neural and physiological mechanisms in the development of stress-related conditions remains at an early stage (Herbert, 1997). In particular, we remain largely ignorant of why one person develops one illness (e.g. depression) rather than another (e.g. coronary ischaemia), and why some are susceptible whilst others seem resilient.

ACKNOWLEDGEMENTS

I am grateful to Gillian Barker for secretarial help. The work of my laboratory is supported by grants from the Wellcome Trust, Medical Research Council (MRC) and the Biotechnology and Biological Sciences Research Council (BBSRC).

REFERENCES

Adolphs, R., Tranel, D., Damasio, H. and Damasio, A.R. (1995). Fear and the human amygdala. *Journal of Neuroscience*, **15**, 5879–5891.

Andreae, L.C. and Herbert, J. (1993). Expression of *c-fos* in restricted areas of the basal forebrain and brainstem following single or combined intraventricular infusions of vasopressin and corticotropin-releasing factor. *Neuroscience*, **53**, 735–48

Arnold, F.J.L., de Lucas Bueno, M., Shiers, H., Hancock, D.C., Evan, G.I. and Herbert, J. (1992). Expression of *c-fos* in regions of the basal limbic forebrain following intra-cerebroventricular corticotropin-releasing factor (CRF) in unstressed or stressed male rats. *Neuroscience*, **51**, 377–390.

Berridge, C.W. and Dunn, A.J. (1989). Restraint-stress-induced changes in exploratory behavior appear to be mediated by norepinephrine-stimulated release of CRF. *Journal of Neuroscience*, **9**, 3513–3521.

Brown, G.W. and Harris, T.O. (Eds) (1989). *Life Events and Illness*. London: Unwin Hyman.

Campeau, S. and Davis, M. (1995). Involvement of subcortical and cortical afferents to the lateral nucleus of the amygdala in fear conditioning measured with fear-potentiated startle in rats trained concurrently with auditory and visual conditioned stimuli. *Journal of Neuroscience*, **15**, 2312–2327.

Campeau, S., Hayward, M.D., Hope, B.T., Rosen, J.B., Nestler, E.J. and Davis, M. (1991). Induction of the c-fos proto-oncogene in rat amygdala during unconditioned and conditioned fear. *Brain Research*, **565**, 349–352.

Cole, B.J., Cador, M., Stinus, L., Rivier, J., Vale, W., Koob, G.F. and Le Moal, M. (1990). Central administration of a CRF antagonist blocks the development of stress-induced behavioral sensitisation. *Brain Research*, **512**, 343–346.

Davidson, R.J. (1992). Anterior cerebral asymmetry and the nature of emotion. *Brain and Cognition*, **20**, 125–151.

De Goeij, D.C.E., Kvetnansky, R., Whitnall, M.H., Jesova, D., Berkenbosch, F. and Tilders, F.J.H. (1991) Repeated stress-induced activation of corticotropinreleasing factor neurons enhances vasopressin stores and colocalization with corticotropin-releasing factor in the median eminence of rats. *Neuroendocrinology*, **53**, 150–159.

Eberhart, J.A., Keverne, E.B. and Meller, R.E. (1980) Social influences on plasma testosterone in male talapoin monkeys. *Hormonal Behaviour*, **14**, 247–266.

Eberhart, J.A.,Yodyingyuad, U. and Keverne, E.B. (1985) Social subordination in male talapoin monkeys lowers sexual behaviour in the absence of dominants. *Physiology and Behavior*, **35**, 673–678.

Elkabir, D.R., Wyatt, M.E., Vellucci, S.V. and Herbert, J. (1990). The effects of separate or combined infusions of corticotropin-releasing factor and vasopressin either intraventricularly or into the amygdala on aggressive and investigative behaviour in the rat. *Regul. Peptides*, **28**, 199–214.

Fitzsimons, J.T. (1998) Angiotensin, thirst and sodium appetite. *Physiological Review*, **78**, 583–686.

Gebarski, S.S., Arbor, A., Starkman, M.N., Berent, S. and Schteingart, D.E. (1996) Cushings syndrome: correlation of hippocampal formation and caudate head volume with cognitive dysfunction and cortisol levels. *Radiology*, **201**, 26.

Gillies, G.E., Linton, E.A. and Lowry, P.J. (1982). Corticotropin-releasing activity of the new CRF is potentiated several times by vasopressin. *Nature*, **299**: 355–357.

Goodyer, I.M., Herbert, J., Altham, P.M.E., Pearson, J., Secher, S.M. and Shiers, H.M. (1996). Adrenal secretion during major depression in 8 to 16 year olds. I. Altered diurnal rhythms in salivary cortisol and dehydroepiandrosterone (DHEA) at presentation. *Psychological Medicine*, **26**, 245–256.

Gurvits, T.V., Shenton, M.E. and Hokama, H. (1996) Magnetic resonance imaging study of hippocampal volume in chronic, combat-related posttraumatic stress disorder. *Biological Psychiatry*, **49**, 1091–1099.

Herbert, J., Forsling, M.L., Howes, S.R., Stacey, P.M. and Shiers, H.M. (1992). Regional expression of *c-fos* antigen in the basal forebrain following intraventricular infusions of angiotensin and its modulation by drinking either water or saline. *Neuroscience*, **51**, 867–882.

Herbert, J. (1993). Peptides in the limbic system: neurochemical codes for coordinated adaptive responses to behavioral and physiological demand. *Progress in Neurobiology*, **41**, 723–791.

Herbert, J. (1996). Sexuality, stress, and the chemical architecture of the brain. *Annual Review of Sex Research*, **7**, 1–43.

Herbert, J. (1997). Stress, the brain and mental illness. *British Medical Journal*, **315**, 530–535.

Hughes, A.M., Everitt, B.J. and Herbert, J. (1987) Selective effects of β-endorphin infused into the hypothalamus, preoptic area and bed nucleus of the stria terminalis. *Neuroscience*, **23**, 1063–1073.

Kagan, J. and Schulkin, J. (1995) On the concepts of fear. *Harvard Review of Psychology*, **3**, 231–234

Kelly, W.F., Checkley, S.A., Bender, D.A. and Mashiter, K. (1983). Cushing's syndrome and depression: a prospective study of 26 patients. *British Journal of Psychiatry*, **142**, 16–19.

Kiecolt-Glaser, J.K., Glaser, R., Cacioppo, J.T., MacCallum, R.C., Snydersmith, M., Kim, C. and Malarkey, W.B. (1997). Marital conflict in older adults: endocrinological and immunological correlates. *Psychosomatic Medicine*, **59**(4), 339–349.

Kimonides, V., Khatibi, N., Svendsen, C.N., Sofroniew, M.V. and Herbert, J. (1998). Dehydroepiandrosterone (DHEA) and DHEA-sulfate protect hippocampal neurons against excitatory amino-acid-induced neurotoxicity. *Proceedings of the National Academy of Science, USA*, **95**, 1852–1857.

Krettek, J.E. and Price, J.L. (1976) Amygdaloid projections to subcortical structures within the basal forebrain and brainstem in the rat and cat. *Journal of Comparataive Neurology*, **178**, 225–254.

LeDoux, J.E. (1994) The amygdala: contributions to fear and stress. *Seminars in the Neurosciences*, **6**, 231–237.

Lewis, D.A. and Smith, R.E. (1983) Steroid-induced psychiatric syndromes. *Journal of Affective Disorders*, **5**, 319–332.

Light, K.C., Kothandapani, R.V. and Allen, M.T. (1998). Enhanced cardiovascular and catecholamine responses in women with depressive symptoms. *International Journal of Psychophysiology*, **28**(2), 157–166.

Luecken, L.J., Suarez, E.C., Kuhn, C.M., Barefoot, J.C., Blumenthal, J.A., Siegler, I.C. and Williams, R.B. (1997). Stress in employed women: impact of marital status and children at home on neurohormone output and home strain. *Psychosomatic Medicine*, **59**(4), 352–359.

Luria, A.R. (1980). *Higher Cortical Functions in Man*. New York: Basic Books.

Ma, X.M. and Lightman, S.L. (1998). The arginine vasopressin and corticotrophin-releasing hormone gene transcription responses to varied frequencies of repeated stress in rats. *Journal of Physiology*, **510**(2), 605–614.

Magarinos, A.M. and McEwen, B.S. (1995). Stress-induced atrophy of apical dendrites of hippocampal CA3c neurons: comparison of stressors. *Neuroscience*, **69**, 83–88.

Maren, S. and Fanselow, M.S. (1996). The amygdala and fear conditioning: has the nut been cracked? *Neuron*, **16**, 237–240.

Martensz, N.D., Vellucci, S.V., Fuller, L.M, Everitt, B.J., Keverne, E.B. and Herbert, J. (1987). Relation between aggressive behaviour and circadian rhythms in cortisol and testosterone in social groups of talapoin monkeys. *Journal of Endocrinology*, **115**, 107–120.

Martinez, M., Phillips, P.J. and Herbert, J. (1998). Adaptation in patterns of *c-fos* expression in the brain associated with exposure to either single or repeated social stress in male rats. *European Journal of Neuroscience*, **10**, 20–33.

Mason, J.W. (1972). Organisation of psychoendocrine mechanisms. In N.S. Greenfield and R.A. Sternbach (eds) *Handbook of Psychophysiology* (3–91). New York: Holt, Rinehart & Winston.

Monnikes, H., Schmidt, B.G., Raybould, H.E. and Tache, Y. (1992) CRF in the paraventricular nucleus mediates gastric and colonic motor response to restraint stress. *American Journal Physiology*, **262**, G137-G143.

Nemeroff, C.B., Widerlov, E., Bissette, G., Wallcus, H., Karlsson, I., Kilts, C.S., Loosen, P.T., and Vale, W. (1984). Elevated concentration of CSF corticotropin-releasing factor-like immunoreactivity in depressed patients. *Science*, **226**, 1342–1344.

Paykel, E.S. and Cooper, Z. (1992). Life events and social stress. In E.S. Paykel (Ed.) *Handbook of Affective Disorders*, 2nd edn, pp. 149–170. Edinburgh: Churchill-Livingstone.

Peters, M.L., Godaert, G.L.R., Ballieux, R.E., van Vliet, M., Willemsen, J.J., Sweep, F.C. and Heijnen, C.J. (1998) Cardiovascular and endocrine responses to experimental stress: effect of mental effort and controllability. *Psychoneuroendocrinology*, **23**, 1–17.

Pike, J.L., Smith, T.L., Hauger, R.L., Nicassio, P.M., Patterson, T.L., McLintick, J., Costlow, C. and Irwin, M.R. (1997). Chronic stress alters sympathetic, neuroendocrine and immune responsivity to an acute psychological stressor in humans. *Psychosomatic Medicine*, **59**, 447–457.

Porter, N.M. and Landfield, P.W. (1998) Stress hormones and brain aging: adding injury to insult? *Nature Neuroscience*, **1**, 3–4.

Price, J.L., Russchen, F.T. and Amaral, D.G. (1987). The limbic region. II: the amygdaloid complex. In A. Bjorklund, T. Hokfelt and L.W. Swanson (Eds) *Handbook of Chemical Neuroanatomy,* **Vol. 5**, pp. 279–388. Amsterdam: Elsevier.

Roozendaal, B., Koolhaas, J.M. and Bohus, B. (1990). Differential effects of lesioning of the central amygdala on the bradycardiac and behavioral response of the rat in relation to conditioned social and solitary stress. *Behavioral Brain Research*. **41**, 39–48.

Roozendaal, B., Koolhaas, J.M. and Bohus, B. (1996). Central amygdaloid involvement in neuroendocrine correlates of conditioned stress responses. *Journal of Neuroendocrinology*, **4**, 483–489.

Roth-Isigkeit, A., Brechmann, J., Dibbelt, L., Sievers, H.H., Raasch, W. and Schmucker, P. (1998). Persistent endocrine stress response in patients undergoing cardiac surgery. *Journal of Endocrinological Investigation*, **21**(1), 12–19.

Sapolsky, R.M. (1986). Stress-induced elevations of testosterone concentrations in high ranking baboons: role of catecholamines. *Endocrinology*, **118**, 1630–1635.

Sapolsky R.M. (1996). Stress, glucocorticoids, and damage to the nervous system: the current state of confusion. *Stress*, **1**, 1–19.

Selye, H. (1978). *The Stress of Life*. New York: McGraw-Hill.

Sheline, Y.I., Wang, P.O., Gado, M.H., Csernansky, J.G., Vannier, M.W. (1996). Hippocampal atrophy in recurrent major depression. *Proceedings of the National Academy of Science, USA*, **93**, 3908–3913.

Southwick, S.M., Morgan, C.A. Bremner, A.D., Grillon, C.G., Krystal, J.H., Nagy, L.M. and Charney, D.S. (1997). Noradrenergic alterations in posttraumatic stress disorder. *Annals of the New York Academy of Sciences*, **821**, 125–141.

Suarez, E.C., Kuhn, C.M., Schanberg, S.M., Williams, R.B. and Zimmermann, E.A. (1998). Neuroendocrine, cardiovascular, and emotional responses of hostile men: the role of interpersonal challenge. *Psychosomatic Medicine*, **60**(1), 78–88.

Thatcher-Britton, K., Lee, G., Vale, W., Rivier, J. and Koob, G.F. (1986). Corticotropin-releasing factor (CRF) receptor antagonist blocks activating and "anxiogenic" actions of CRF in the rat. *Brain Research*, **369**, 303–306.

Uno, H., Tarara, R., Else, J.G., Suleman, M.A. and Sapolsky, R.M. (1989). Hippocampal damage associated with prolonged and fatal stress in primates. *Journal of Neuroscience*, **9**, 1705–1711.

Wolkowitz, O.M. (1994). Prospective controlled-studies of the behavioral and biological effects of exogenous corticosteroids. *Psychoneuroendocrinology*, **19**, 233–255.

Yehuda,R,, Siever, L.J., Teicher, M.H., Levengood, R.A., Gerber, D.K., Schmeidler, J. and Yang, R.K. (1998). Plasma norepinephrine and 3-methoxy-4-hydroxyphenylglycol concentrations and severity of depression in combat post traumatic stress disorder and major depressive disorder. *Biological Psychiatry*, **44**(1), 56–63.

Yodyingyuad, U., Eberhart, J.A. and Keverne, E.B. (1982). Effects of rank and novel females on behaviour and hormones in male talapoin monkeys. *Physiology and Behavior*, **28**, 995–1005.

5

FALLIBILITY, UNCERTAINTY AND THE IMPACT OF MISTAKES AND LITIGATION

Charles Vincent

Doctors and other health professionals face long hours and daily encounters with sick and dying people, often working in a difficult and sometimes chaotic environment. The expectations of patients and relatives cannot always be met. There is, for instance, often a wish for certainty when medical knowledge can only offer an approximation or overall probability of recovery (McCue, 1982). In many specialties the stress inherent in the job is compounded by a work ethic that is incompatible with a satisfying life outside medicine. None of this is to deny that the work and relationships with both patients and colleagues can be immensely rewarding, but the rewards are tempered to an unusual extent by a variety of adverse effects on health professionals.

The main sources of stress will be briefly described, but this chapter is primarily concerned with the impact of errors and mistakes, and the events that follow them. Human beings make frequent errors and misjudgements in every sphere of activity, but some environments are less forgiving of error than others. Errors in academia, law or architecture, for instance, can often be remedied with an apology or a cheque. Those in medicine, aviation, oil and chemical industries may have severe or even

Stress in Health Professionals. Edited by Jenny Firth-Cozens and Roy L. Payne
© 1999 John Wiley & Sons Ltd

catastrophic consequences. This is not to say that the errors of doctors or pilots are more reprehensible, only that they bear a greater burden because their errors have greater consequences. All these observations apply to some degree to other health professionals, but the limited research in this area is almost entirely restricted to doctors. There is a large literature on nursing medication errors, for instance, but, with some exceptions, little research on the impact of errors on nurses (Meurier et al., 1997).

SOURCES OF STRESS IN MEDICAL PRACTICE

The most obvious, and most frequently cited sources of stress in medicine, particularly for young doctors, are long hours and excessive workload, which in turn are seen as impeding good care (Firth-Cozens, 1993; McKee and Black, 1992). In a qualitative questionnaire study, Firth-Cozens and Greenhalgh (1997) found that 82 of a sample of 225 hospital doctors and general practitioners reported recent incidents where they considered that symptoms of stress had negatively affected patient care. Half of these incidents led to lowered standards of care, including two patient deaths.

However, long hours are not the only, or even the main, source of stress for many. When asked to describe a recent stressful event British junior doctors singled out making mistakes, together with dealing with death and dying, relationships with senior doctors and overwork (Firth-Cozens, 1987). When Mizrahi (1984) asked young interns "What were your most memorable experiences during training?", 21% of the replies concerned actual or potential mistakes. In addition, he found that serious and even fatal mistakes were made by half of the new interns he interviewed in the first two months of their jobs.

The many stressors in doctors' lives combine to influence high levels of depression, alcohol abuse and suicide in doctors (see Chapter 6, this volume). Depression and the other effects of stress affect performance in a variety of ways, increasing the risk of error, reducing confidence and self-esteem which may in turn lead to deeper depression in a vicious spiral. Although treated separately here, fallibility and mistakes are therefore, intimately linked with other stressors.

THE NATURE OF HUMAN ERROR

Errors are commonly divided into two broad categories: those where the plan is adequate but the action is not as intended (termed slips, lapses, or trips) and those where the action may be correct, but the plan is inadequate. The latter are failures of intention, termed mistakes (Reason, 1990). There are many varieties of medical error and no absolute dividing line between error and correct performance. Some departures from procedures, for instance incorrect drug dosages, are clear-cut errors. Other types of mismanagement may appear correct at the time, yet later be seen to be erroneous. Others still may be more strongly grounded in genuine uncertainty, being a form of what Gorowitz and MacIntyre (1976) have termed "necessary fallibility". In brief, necessary fallibility stems from their view of medicine as a "science of particulars", in which every patient presents uniquely. For example, where a disease presents in an extreme form, clinicians can easily make an incorrect diagnosis. However, this is due primarily to the presentation of the disease, rather than the personal fallibility of the clinician. Few of these various types of error can be simply attributed to individual fallibility, and still less are they blameworthy or negligent (in the sense of a clear departure from standard care which caused harm).

Irrespective of how errors are defined, it is clear that in medicine they are extremely common. Studies of the accuracy of tests and clinical procedures suggest that high rates of error have been found in detecting the clinical signs of cyanosis, interpreting electrocardiograms and radiographs, taking a history and assessing biopsy specimens in the laboratory. Even basic skills such as resuscitation have been found to fall well short of the expected standard (Vincent, 1989). The causes of such errors are numerous and include an incomplete or erroneous knowledge base, inattentiveness, procedural inaccuracies, premature closure, faulty reasoning and a proneness of human cognition to bias and a variety of environmental and organisational factors (see below). Errors are made for many reasons, most not in control of the individual, and to equate error automatically with incompetence or irresponsibility is, from a psychological perspective, ridiculous.

Most mistakes cause no harm to patients and as such go unnoticed by the patient, the family, the clinician and colleagues. However, considerable numbers of patients are actually harmed by their treatment. The Harvard study found that adverse events, occasions on which patients are unintentionally harmed by treatment, occurred in almost 4% of admissions in New York State. For 70% of patients the resulting disability was slight or short-lived, but in 7% it was permanent and 14% of patients died in part as a result of their treatment (Brennan et al., 1991). Serious harm therefore came to approximately 1% of patients admitted to hospital. Similar findings have recently been reported from studies carried out in Colorado and Utah in 1992 (Vincent, 1997). An Australian study has revealed that 16.6% of admissions resulted in an adverse event, of which half were considered preventable (Wilson *et al.*, 1995); and a more recent American observational study found that 45% of patients experienced some mismanagement during their hospital stay and that 17% suffered events that led to a longer hospital stay or more serious problems (Andrews *et al.*, 1997). These events also involve a huge personal cost to the people involved, both patients and staff. Many patients suffer increased pain, disability and psychological trauma, often compounded by a protracted, adversarial legal process (Vincent *et al.*, 1993).

THE CAUSES OF ADVERSE EVENTS

The causes of adverse events are complex. Many could not have been prevented. Some are the result of genuine uncertainty in diagnosis and decision making. Even where errors have occurred, they are often only part of a chain of events inseparable from a web of organisational background causes. Seldom, after close analysis, is it possible to lay the blame for an adverse outcome solely at the door of one individual, however tempting this may be.

Analyses of accidents in medicine and elsewhere have led to a much broader understanding of accident causation, with less focus on the individual unsafe acts or omissions and more on the work environment—pre-existing organisational factors that provide the conditions in which errors occur (Cook and Woods, 1994; Cooper *et al.*, 1984; Vincent and Bark, 1995). In medicine the root causes of adverse events may lie in factors such as communication and supervision problems, excessive workload, educational and training deficiencies, the use of locums and so on. Junior doctors, for instance, may find themselves forced to deal with events that are well beyond their competence. From this perspective the junior doctor in the front line may be the inheritor of others' mistakes and deficiencies. For them to then take responsibility and shoulder all the blame may be both unwarranted and personally damaging. Vincent (1997) suggests that, after serious incidents, the first question should be "What does this tell us about our system?", and only then "What does this tell us about this individual?". This approach puts a very different perspective on responsibility and blame for adverse outcomes (which is not to deny that blame is perfectly appropriate in the case of persistent, intentional neglect of duty).

ATTITUDES TO ERROR

In a landmark paper on error in medicine, Leape (1994) has speculated as to why high error rates in medicine have not stimulated more concern and efforts at error prevention. One reason may be a lack of awareness of the problem since most errors do not lead to harm, and serious adverse events are not part of the everyday experience of clinicians but are perceived as isolated and unusual events. However, Leape argues that the most important reason is that clinicians have difficulty dealing with error when it does occur, and that this difficulty is grounded in the culture of medical practice:

> *Physicians are socialised in medical school and residency to strive for error-free practice. There is a powerful emphasis on perfection, both in diagnosis and treatment. In everyday hospital practice, the message is equally clear: mistakes are unacceptable. Physicians are expected to function without error, an expectation that physicians translate into the need to be infallible. One result is that physicians, not unlike test pilots, come to view an error as a failure of character—you weren't careful, you didn't try hard enough. This kind of thinking lies behind a common reaction by clinicians: "How can there be an error without negligence."*
> (Leape, 1994)

Leape goes on to argue that role models in medical education reinforce the idea of infallibility, leading in turn to a pressure for intellectual dishonesty, and errors rarely being openly discussed. McIntyre and Popper (1983) go further, arguing that this attitude to error is rooted in a discredited view of the growth of scientific knowledge. According to Popper's philosophy, recognition of error lies at the heart of scientific and medical progress, and McIntyre and Popper argue powerfully for a new critical attitude in medicine, a new ethic centred on an explicit recognition of fallibility and error.

All clinicians recognise the inevitability (though perhaps not the frequency) of error. However, this seldom carries over into open recognition and discussion, and still less into research on error. There is therefore a curious, and in some ways paradoxical, clash of beliefs. On the one hand, we have an enterprise fraught with uncertainty, where knowledge is inadequate and actions are bound to be imperfect if not erroneous. On the other hand, those working in this environment foster a culture of perfection in which errors are not tolerated and in which a strong sense of personal responsibility both for errors and outcome is expected. The strong sense of responsibility is in many ways appropriate and necessary. However, there is a clash between reality and culture, and between reality and the expectations of both patients and clinicians. With this background it is not surprising that mistakes are hard to deal with, particularly when so much else is at stake in terms of human suffering.

THE IMPACT OF MISTAKES

Occasional papers on mistakes are evident in the medical literature, but there is no sustained body of research into their impact. Those that have tried to bring the subject into the open have not always fared well at the hands of their colleagues. For instance, Hilfiker (1984) argued that "We see the horror of our own mistakes, yet we are given no permission to deal with their enormous emotional impact . . . The medical profession simply has no place for its mistakes." This paper drew some supportive correspondence, but also comments such as "This neurotic piece has no place in the New England Journal of Medicine" (Anderson, 1984). Hilfiker hoped that others would follow his example and write about their own errors, but was apparently disappointed that progress was slow thereafter (Ely, 1996).

The impact of mistakes was explored in interviews with 11 doctors by Christensen and colleagues (1992). Although this small study did not assess the overall importance of mistakes, a number of very important themes are discussed, in particular: the ubiquity of mistakes in clinical practice; the infrequency of self-disclosure about mistakes to colleagues, friends and family; the degree of emotional impact on the physician, so that some mistakes were remembered in great detail even after several years; and the influence of beliefs about personal responsibility and medical practice. A variety of mistakes were discussed, all with serious outcomes including four deaths. All were affected to some degree, but four clinicians described intense agony or anguish as the reality of the mistake had sunk in.

> I was really shaken. My whole feelings of self-worth and abilities were basically profoundly shaken.

> I was appalled and devastated that I had done this to somebody.

> My great fear was that I had missed something, and then there was a sense of panic.

> It was hard to concentrate on anything else I was doing because I was so worried about what was happening, so I guess that would be anxiety. I felt guilty, sad, had trouble sleeping, wondering what was going on.

After the initial shock the clinicians had a variety of reactions that had lasted from several days to several months. Some of the feelings of fear, guilt, anger, embarrassment and humiliation were unresolved at the time of the interview, even a year after the mistake. A few reported symptoms of depression, including disturbances in appetite, sleep and concentration. Fears related to concerns for the patient's welfare, litigation and colleagues' discovery of their "incompetence", and these fears prevented some from airing their feelings with other professionals. For others there was a cynicism about the tendency of other physicians to minimise the mistake or to restrict discussion to the problem-solving aspects of the case, ignoring the emotional concerns. In an experimental study with family physicians Newman (1996) found that almost all clinicians stated a need for support after a serious error, but only one-third were willing to provide it unconditionally. Clinicians needed the emotional support and professional reaffirmation, but their culture did not often permit such open discussions.

The Christensen study is rich in detail, but confined to a small sample of potentially untypical individuals. Wu and colleagues (1991), however, sent questionnaires to 254 interns in the USA asking the respondents to describe the most significant mistake in patient care they had made in the last year, which had serious or potentially serious consequences for the patient. Almost all the errors had serious outcomes and almost a third involved a death. Wu found that accepting responsibility for the error was most likely to result in constructive changes in practice (i.e. learning from the error), though accepting responsibility was also associated with higher levels of distress.

House officers reported discussing the mistake with the supervisory clinician in only 54% of cases, though 88% of mistakes were discussed with another clinician, and 58% with a non-medical person. Only 24% of mistakes were discussed with the patient or patient's family. Feelings of remorse, anger, guilt and inadequacy were common. Over a quarter of house officers feared negative repercussions from the mistake. A few reported persistent negative reactions. "This case has made me very nervous about clinical medicine. I worry now about all febrile patients since they may be on the verge of sepsis." For another house officer, a missed diagnosis made him reject a career in subspecialties that involve "a lot of data collection and uncertainty". This echoes the experience of Carlo Fonsecka (1996) who recounted the personal impact of mistakes in a remarkable personal paper that began "Error free patient care is the ideal standard but in reality unattainable. I am conscious of having made five fatal mistakes during the past 36 years." Fonsecka wrote that, with hindsight, he believes that the impact of the first case was so great that he no longer felt able to carry on with clinical work and turned eventually to a laboratory-based career.

Clearly only a small proportion of errors are so traumatic. What singles out a mistake as being traumatic? There is little research on this issue, but some ideas can be put forward. First, and most obviously, the outcome will be severe. Hindsight bias applies in this area, in that retrospective judgements of substandard care with a poor outcome are harsher than those of the same care with an acceptable outcome (Caplan *et al.*, 1988; Caplan *et al.*, 1991). Second, it will be a clear departure from the clinician's usual practice, rather than an instance of "necessary fallibility" in a genuinely uncertain situation. Third, there will at least the potential for criticism from others. Fourth, a close involvement with the patient or family. For instance psychologists or psychiatrists may find the suicide of a patient very hard to face if there has been a long therapeutic relationship. For a highly self-critical person, errors and mistakes will be particularly disturbing, causing further stress which may in turn make him or her more likely to make mistakes. Firth-Cozens (1997) has found that a tendency to self-criticism—itself rooted in earlier relationships—is predictive of later stress and finds an echo in relationships with senior colleagues.

THE IMPACT OF COMPLAINTS AND LITIGATION

The impact of errors and mistakes is compounded and deepened when complaints or litigation follow. The relationship between the patient and the health professional, whether doctor, nurse or other professional, has changed profoundly over the past 20 years. Patients demand much more of the doctor or nurse, are more likely to question his or her skills, and are considerably less forgiving when their own expectations of outcome are not fulfilled, whether or not this is the result of error, accident or malpractice. As the public perception has changed, patients have become more forceful in criticising professionals, and are more likely to resort to litigation. Media attention has also made the public much more aware of the potential for harm as well as benefit from medical treatment.

The experience of being sued in a prolonged and difficult case is documented in Charles and Kennedy's (1985) book, *Defendant: A Psychiatrist on Trial for Medical Malpractice*:

> *My first feelings after being charged with medical malpractice were being utterly alone. Suddenly, I felt isolated from my colleagues and patients. Since then I have learned in the course of my own suit and trial and in the research I have conducted, that this feeling of aloneness is not at all unusual, that almost every physician accused of being negligent has a similar reaction. I also understand that what I experienced during the five year span of my case—that it swallowed up my life completely, demanded constant attention and study, multiplied tensions and strain, generated a pattern of broken sleep and anxiety because I felt my integrity as a person and a physician had been damaged and might be permanently lost—are the common reactions of most doctors accused of negligence. (Charles and Kennedy, 1985)*

There is little research on the impact of complaints, but a number of studies of the effects of litigation. Depression, anger, shame and loss of confidence are common responses (Charles *et al.*, 1985; Martin *et al.*, 1991; Bark *et al.*, 1997). Charles *et al.* (1985) found that sued physicians were more likely to report that they were likely to stop seeing certain types of patients, think of retiring early and discourage their children from entering medicine. Older physicians, however, have been found to be less affected and more able to put litigation into perspective, as a job hazard rather than an indictment of their ability (Martin *et al.*, 1991).

In a development of Charles's work, Shapiro *et al.* (1989) surveyed 171 matched pairs of sued physicians and their patients who were taking action together with a sample of 100 non-sued physicians. Sued physicians stated that they found the practice of medicine less rewarding and satisfying after legal action. Bark *et al.* (1997), in a survey of over 100 British hospital consultants and senior registrars, examined both the impact of litigation on British clinicians and also their suggestions for support and assistance. Support from friends, colleagues, management and outside professionals was seen as very important. There were some embittered and angry comments about the lack of personal support from managers with descriptions of unfair criticism, judgement and witch hunting. Support groups, counselling, nominated mentors and legal advice within the hospital system were often proposed, both as an information resource and for moral support. Most considered, however, that the threat of litigation had led to attempts to improve communication with patients and staff and to keep better records.

Shapiro *et al.* (1989) found that clinicians who were more involved with their patients experienced more anger, tension and depression and sense of defeat as a result of legal action, than those who were less involved. Similarly, patients who had honest initial relationships with their doctors reported the strongest negative feelings as a result of litigation. The study also suggested that malpractice litigation is often preceded by difficulties in the relationship. Two-thirds of sued doctors thought that they had been open and honest with their patients, but only one-third of patients agreed. Recent studies of obstetricians with high levels of litigation, compared with colleagues, suggest that those with litigation histories are distinguished not by the quality of their care, but by different attitudes, insensitivity, and poorer communication skills (Entman *et al.*, 1994; Hickson *et al.*, 1994).

WHAT CAN BE DONE?

There is clearly a need to address the various sources of stress experienced by health professionals. Work needs to be restructured to offer better support and sleep patterns, and, if possible, shorter hours. Depression, anxiety and alcohol abuse can be treated by specialist job-related counselling and psychotherapy, shown to both reduce symptoms and change job attitudes in a positive direction (Firth-Cozens, 1993). Committed training is needed for undergraduates in ways to cope with the stressors which are inevitable. However, there are also specific measures that could be taken which would reduce the impact of stress due to fallibility, mistakes and their consequences.

Potential for error must be acknowledged

The potential for error in medicine, as in other activities, needs to be recognised and openly acknowledged. In novel situations, and at times of stress and uncertainty, the probability of slips and mistakes inevitably increases, no matter how conscientious the clinician (Reason, 1990). Error prevention usually involves exhortation, training or disciplinary measures all directed at the individual (Leape, 1994). Personal motivation and discipline are supposed to overcome biological and psychological constraints. However, people do not intend to make errors and it is often pointless to chastise them for doing so. Rather we must move towards a systems approach of examining why events and adverse events occur (Leape, 1997).

Education about the ubiquity of error, its causes and likely consequences, would bring a more realistic attitude and constructive approach. It should also be possible to identify those students who may be vulnerable to excessive reactions to errors—for example, those in whom tutors see signs of self-blame in clinical discussions. High self-criticism is a way of thinking, a cognitive style in which self blame occurs whenever things go wrong; it can therefore be changed by teaching students how to allocate responsibility less destructively (Firth-Cozens, 1997).

Education about medical law and the legal process

Part of the horror of a complaint or threat of litigation lies, for young clinicians at least, simply in ignorance of what is involved. They may, for instance, believe that they will be faced with trial by jury. Education in legal matters for all staff, together with specific information about the likely course of any complaint or claim, can reduce a great deal of unnecessary distress. As well as providing important guidance about what the law requires on such matters as confidentiality, consent and decisions to treat or withdraw treatment (Genn, 1995), hospital solicitors may be willing to organise teaching sessions for specified groups of staff, or to provide an expert who can attend an occasional seminar. Many doctors act as experts in negligence cases and therefore have considerable experience of the litigation process. Through their examination of material relating to negligence claims they have knowledge about the kinds of actions that lead to allegations of negligence in their particular specialty and therefore represent an important educative resource for their peers and for the junior staff. Through their experience of litigation procedures they can communicate practical information about what happens in the course of a negligence action (Hirst, 1996).

Formal support and access to confidential counselling

Not everyone needs support when faced with a complaint or litigation, but it does help to know that someone is available to provide a sympathetic ear. The range of potential support extends from a quiet word in a corridor to the offer of extended psychotherapy. Because the range is so wide, the choice of intensity must be left to the individual concerned, who should feel free to ask for a greater or lesser degree of involvement as time goes on. Managers tempted to provide "stress counselling", especially from paid sources outside the organisation, should remember that support from immediate colleagues is usually much more welcome and appropriate, and that some degree of anxiety is normal in times of stress. People are resilient, but anyone may be vulnerable, because of personality, position or circumstance, to distressingly severe reactions. Some hospitals employ recently retired consultants as mentors. A link with a psychiatrist or psychologist, perhaps outside the hospital trust, might also be useful when the strain is severe or prolonged, as occurs when a member of staff feels responsible for a serious injury or death (Hirst, 1996).

Communication skills training

When things go wrong and a patient is harmed or disturbed in some way it is vital, for all concerned that an explanation is given, an apology where appropriate, and remedial treatment and counselling instituted. Facing a patient harmed by treatment, or the patient's naturally distressed and angry relatives, is a particularly difficult clinical situation for which little guidance or training is available. A final important area, for both patients and staff, is the provision of training in communication skills for coping with, and helping, dissatisfied, distressed or injured patients and their relatives.

Some litigation and many formal complaints could probably be avoided by a sensitive initial response to complaints or incidents in which patients have been harmed (Vincent et al., 1994). When formal complaints or litigation have been initiated, it may still be helpful for the risk management team to negotiate a settlement which does not involve a protracted legal process with all the attendant expense and strain on both patients and staff.

Agreed policy on openness with injured patients

The openness and sensitivity of individual clinicians will, however, be thoroughly and fatally undermined if there is not a collaborative approach between clinicians and management with a basic strategy agreed by the hospital trust board. Early intervention with injured patients is only feasible if backed by a management policy that encourages doctors to be open with patients about mistakes that have been made. Some doctors are still torn between their own desire for a more open stance and the more cautious approach that they perceive to be demanded, rightly or wrongly, by managers and the defence societies. This can turn an already very difficult situation into a conflict that is traumatic for staff and patient alike. This brings home the extent to which a different approach to error and adverse events on the part of clinicians must be mirrored by a similar shift in attitudes on the part of managers, lawyers, and indeed patients and relatives.

The most important change that is needed is a move towards a less confrontational, adversarial approach to resolving disputes and compensation issues. In Britain at least there have been very encouraging and positive changes over the last ten years. In the early 1980s many plaintiff and defendant lawyers fought cases with little thought of the effect on the other side's clients; doctor and patient were adversaries in a contest. Now, in contrast, representatives from all professions and groups are making major efforts to move towards a more humane and rational approach. Medical injury and the associated human suffering are being openly acknowledged on all sides and it is not unreasonable to hope that this new openness will gradually bring benefits to staff and patients alike.

REFERENCES

Anderson, M. (1984). Facing our mistakes. *New England Journal of Medicine*, **310**, 1676.

Andrews, L.B., Stocking, C., Krizek, T., Gottlieb, L., Krizek, C., Vargish, T. and Siegler, M. (1997). An alternative strategy for studying adverse events in medical care. *Lancet*, **349**, 309–313.

Bark, P., Vincent, C., Olivieri, L. and Jones, A. (1997). Impact of litigation on senior clinicians: implications for risk management. *Quality in Health Care*, **6**, 7–13.

Brennan, T.A., Leape, L.L., Laird, N.M., Hebert, L., Localio, A.R., Lawthers, A.G., Newhouse, J.P., Weiler, P.C. and Hiatt, H.H. (1991). Incidence of adverse events and negligence in hospitalized patients. *New England Journal of Medicine*, **324**(6), 370–376.
Caplan, R.A., Posner, K., Ward, R.J. and Cheney, F.W. (1988). Peer reviewer agreement for major anaesthetic mishaps. *Quality Review Bulletin* (December), 363–368.
Caplan, R.A., Posner, K.L. and Cheney, F.W. (1991). Effect of outcome on physicians' judgements of appropriateness of care. *Journal of the American Medical Association*, **265**, 1957–1960.
Charles, S.C. (1984). A different view of malpractice. *Chicago Medicine*, **87**, 848–850.
Charles, S.C. and Kennedy, E. (1985). *Defendant: A Psychiatrist on Trial for Medical Malpractice*. New York: Free Press.
Charles, S.C., Wilbert, J.R. and Franke, K.J. (1985). Sued and non-sued physicians' self-reported reactions to malpractice litigation. *American Journal of Psychiatry*, **192**(4), 437–440.
Christensen, J.F., Levinson, W. and Dunn, P.M. (1992). The heart of darkness: the impact of perceived mistakes on physicians. *Journal of General Internal Medicine*, **7**, 424–431.
Cook, R.I. and Woods, D.D. (1994). Operating at the sharp end: the complexity of human error. In M.S. Bogner (Ed.) *Human Error in Medicine* (pp. 255–310). Hillsdale, NJ: Erlbaum.
Cooper, J.B., Newbower, R.S. and Kitz, R.J. (1984). An analysis of major errors and equipment failures in anaesthesia management considerations for prevention and detection. *Anesthesiology*, **60**, 34–42.
Ely, J.W. (1996). Physicians' mistakes. Will your colleagues offer support? *Archives of Family Medicine*, **5**, 76–77.
Entman, S.S., Glass, C.A., Hickson, G.B., Githens, P.B., Whetten-Goldstein, K. and Sloan, F.A. (1994). The relationship between malpractice claims history and subsequent obstetric care. *Journal of the American Medical Association*, **272**(20), 1588–1591.
Firth-Cozens, J. (1987). Emotional distress in junior house officers. *British Medical Journal*, **295**, 533–536.
Firth-Cozens, J. (1993). Stress, psychological problems and clinical performance. In C.A. Vincent, M. Ennis and & R.J. Audley (Eds) *Medical Accidents* (pp. 131–149). Oxford: Oxford University Press.
Firth-Cozens, J. (1997). Predicting stress in general practitioners: 10 year follow up postal survey. *British Medical Journal*, **315**, 34–35.
Firth-Cozens, J. and Greenhalgh, J. (1997). Doctors' perceptions of the links between stress and lowered clinical care. *Social Science and Medicine*, **44**(7), 1017–1022.
Fonsecka, C. (1996). To err was fatal. *British Medical Journal*, **313**, 1640–1642.
Genn, H. (1995). Supporting staff involved in litigation. In C.A. Vincent (Ed.) *Clinical Risk Management* (pp. 453–472). London: BMJ Publications.
Gorowitz, S. and MacIntyre, A. (1976). Toward a theory of medical fallibility. In H.T. Engelhart and D. Callahan (Eds) *Science, Ethics and Medicine* (pp. 248–274). Hastings-on-Hudson, New York: Hastings Center.
Groves, E.W. (1908). A plea for the uniform registration of operation results. *British Medical Journal*, **2**, 1008–1009.

Hickson, G.B., Clayton, E.W., Entman, S.S., Miller, C.S., Githens, P.B., Whetten-Goldstein, K. and Sloan, F.A. (1994). Obstetricians' prior malpractice experience and patients' satisfaction with care. *Journal of the American Medical Association*, **272**(20), 1583–1587.

Hilfiker, D. (1984). Facing our mistakes. *New England Journal of Medicine*, **310**(2), 118–122.

Hirst, D. (1996). Supporting staff during litigation—managerial aspects. *Clinical Risk*, **2**, 189–194.

Leape, L. (1997). A systems analysis approach to medical error. *Journal of Evaluation in Clinical Practice*, **3**(3), 213–222.

Leape, L.L. (1994). Error in medicine. *Journal of the American Medical Association*, **272**(23), 1851–1857.

Martin, C.A., Wilson, J.F., Siebelman, N.D., Gurley, D.N. and Miller, T.W. (1991). Physician's psychological reactions to malpractice litigation. *Southern Medical Journal*, **84**(11), 1300–1304.

McCue, J.D. (1982). The effects of stress on physicians and their medical practice. *The New England Journal of Medicine*, **306**(8), 458–463.

McIntyre, N. and Popper, K. (1983). The critical attitude in medicine: the need for a new ethics. *British Medical Journal*, **287**, 1919–1923.

McKee, M. and Black, N. (1992). Does the current use of junior doctors in the United Kingdom affect the quality of medical care? *Social Science and Medicine*, **34**(5), 549–558.

Meurier, C.E., Vincent, C.A. and Parmar, D.G. (1997). Learning from errors in nursing practice. *Journal of Advanced Nursing*, **26**, 111–119.

Mizrahi, T. (1984). Managing medical mistakes: ideology, insularity and accountability among internists in training. *Social Science Medicine*, **19**(2), 135–145.

Newman, M.C. (1996). The emotional impact of mistakes on family physicians. *Archives of Family Medicine* **5**, 71–75.

Reason, J.T. (1990). *Human Error*. New York: Cambridge University Press.

Shapiro, R.S., Simpson, D.E., Lawrence, S.L., Talsky, A.M., Sobocinski, K.A. and Schiedermayer, D. L. (1989). A survey of sued and non-sued physicians and suing patients. *Archives of Internal Medicine*, **149**, 2190–2196.

Vincent, C., Young, M. and Phillips, A. (1994). Why do people sue doctors? A study of patients and relatives taking legal action. *The Lancet*, **343** (25 June), 1609–1613.

Vincent, C.A. (1989). Research into medical accidents: a case of negligence? *British Medical Journal*, **299**, 1150–1153.

Vincent, C.A. (1997). Risk, safety and the dark side of quality. *British Medical Journal*, **314**, 1775–6.

Vincent, C.A. and Bark, P. (1995). Accident investigation: discovering why things go wrong. In C.A. Vincent (Ed.) *Clinical Risk Management* (pp. 391–410). London: BMJ Publications.

Vincent, C.A., Pincus, T. and Scurr, J.H. (1993). Patients' experience of surgical accidents. *Quality in Health Care*, **2**, 77–82.

Wilson, R.M., Runciman, W.B., Gibber, R.W., Harrison, B.T., Newby, L. and Hamilton, J.D. (1995). The Quality in Australian Health Care Study. *Medical Journal of Australia*, **163**, 458–471.

Wu, A.W., Folkman, S., McPhee, S.J. and Lo, B. (1991). Do house officers learn from their mistakes? *Journal of the American Medical Association*, **265**(16), 2089–2094.

PART II

THE PROFESSIONS AND THEIR STRESS

6

THE PSYCHOLOGICAL
PROBLEMS OF DOCTORS

Jenny Firth-Cozens

The most tragic thing in the world is a sick doctor, said George Bernard Shaw in *The Doctor's Dilemma*. His opinion was given without the knowledge that, for psychological distress of various kinds, a greater proportion of medical professionals are sick or impaired than is apparent in the rest of the working population. In particular, this takes the form of high levels of stress, depression and alcoholism. This chapter looks at the levels and sources of these problems and suggests a variety of potential interventions to reduce them.

In terms of the general symptoms of stress, as measured by the General Health Questionnaire (Goldberg, 1978), studies show that between 28 and 30% of British doctors are suffering above threshold, compared to 18% of workers employed outside the health profession (Wall *et al.*, 1997). This figure of around 28% has been replicated in a number of studies, and appears to be consistent even at different stages of the career (Firth-Cozens, in press).

Measures of depression levels are not so consistent, probably because of the different means of measurement used in the various studies. However, we know that it accounts for between 21 and 64% of psychiatric admissions in doctors (Rucinski and Cybulska, 1985) and appears to be higher than some other professional groups (Caplan, 1994), with those in the first postgraduate year being particularly at risk (Reuben, 1985; Firth-Cozens, 1987). Reuben followed doctors in their first three years after graduation, assessing them with the Center for Epidemiological Studies

Stress in Health Professionals. Edited by Jenny Firth-Cozens and Roy L. Payne
© 1999 John Wiley & Sons Ltd

Depression Scale monthly. In first year he found 38% depressed at peak times with 29% overall, dropping to 22% in second and 10% in third year.

Women doctors are often reported to be more vulnerable than men to stress and depression, though there are considerable discrepancies in findings both between countries and within them (Gross, 1997). A 10-year longitudinal study of over 300 doctors, begun in their undergraduate years, has shown no differences in stress levels at any time, though women became more depressed than men upon graduation. As more senior doctors, eight years later, there are again no gender differences in stress or depression. However, unlike those in general practice, female hospital doctors are significantly more depressed than male colleagues. This and the finding that, unlike men, student levels of depression are not a predictor of later depression (Brewin and Firth-Cozens, 1997; Firth-Cozens, 1998) appears to indicate that in female doctors there may be more job-related causes of morbidity than in males. It may be that the culture of much of hospital medicine and the lack of female role models for women within certain specialties act to dash hopes of particular career paths, or create extra problems by having to fight one's corner within areas of medicine still reluctant to welcome women. In addition, very few specialties, or even general practice, provide opportunities for a relaxed family life, which may affect women more than men. However, the conflicts between career and family are today seen as equal for men and women (Firth-Cozens, 1995).

There is high co-morbidity between depression and alcoholism, and a study of 100 recovered alcoholic women doctors (Bissel and Skorina, 1987) showed that 73 of them had serious suicidal ideation prior to becoming sober, with 38 making at least one definite suicide attempt. Alcoholism is seen as a particular problem for physicians, as highlighted in a report from the British Medical Association (1998). The extent of the problem is difficult to judge because the doctors concerned, like most alcoholics, are slow to admit to their problem (Brooke et al., 1991), and their colleagues are slow to confront it (Sclare, 1979). In Brooke et al.'s (1991) study of 144 doctors admitted to British units with alcohol and drug problems, some of this abuse was apparent even before entry to medical school, and the latest BMA report suggests that entrants may increasingly begin medicine as addicts or heavy abusers of illegal drugs since young people now begin using them so much earlier. This has certainly been suggested by studies in the USA (Conrad et al., 1988).

Data using SMRs for chronic liver disease and cirrhosis in male doctors, show there is a small excess of deaths over the general population (British Medical Association, 1998). A more detailed look at cirrhotic deaths in Scottish doctors (Harrison and Chick, 1994) concluded that they were also at higher risk than other professionals, especially for those over the age of

45. In my own study, 5% of doctors were scoring in the top category of my scale ("using a lot of alcohol frequently") both in their first postgraduate year and also eight years later as more senior physicians; and individuals' alcohol use over these eight years was highly correlated (0.42, $p<0.001$). Women doctors' current alcohol use, unlike men's, was highly correlated with their stress and depression levels, though it may be that alcohol actually helps coping early on in one's medical career (Khantzian and Mack, 1994), and that the recognition of alcohol-related problems comes later in men than in women. Flaherty and Richman (1993), in an excellent review of the situation in the USA, report that alcohol use actually increases in women students so that it equals male colleagues on graduation, but that alcohol problems increase with age in doctors as a whole, contrary to the trend in the general US population.

Despite these elevated rates of stress, depression and alcohol abuse, there is also evidence that doctors frequently have no general practitioner of their own, that most self-medicate, and that their response to illness is to continue to work (Baldwin et al., 1997a; Pullen et al., 1995). It is clear from this brief review that problems are frequently long-standing, untreated, and appear proportionally higher than in other occupational groups.

THE COSTS TO PATIENT CARE

So much morbidity involves a personal cost to the doctors concerned, but also to patients in terms of lowered care, and to the organisation, in particular in regard to poor performance, patient complaints and litigation. The effects of stress on patient care are usually assessed by the relationship of the number of hours worked or sleep lost to performance on a variety of cognitive tasks (Orton and Gruzelier, 1989). Most studies show that it is the exhaustion that comes from sleep loss which lowers mood as well as performance (Firth-Cozens, 1993). In line with this, the principal attribution for poor care—from general carelessness and irritability through to serious error and even patient death—given by the doctors themselves is tiredness (Firth-Cozens and Greenhalgh, 1997). The worryingly high level of anger and abuse towards patients found in this study is also confirmed by others (McKee and Black, 1992). The costs to patient care of the effects of alcohol abuse are also likely to be high, if unknown. The links between stress, tiredness, alcohol abuse and patient care are well summed up by the comment of a junior anaesthetist: "I am so tired so often that I just want to collapse in a chair and have a few drinks. This causes shaky hands the next day so epidurals, etc., are more difficult" (Firth-Cozens, 1993).

As patients and carers becomes more litigious, the cost to organisations of doctors' exhaustion and its consequences is likely to escalate unless the problem is tackled systematically and vigorously. And it is not only the patients who are now using litigation to redress harm caused by stressors such as inadequate sleep; the first cases of doctors and others successfully suing for the damage done to them by their jobs are proving to be another organisational cost and one which is likely to rise dramatically.

In addition, there are a number of studies which make it clear that doctors who have low job satisfaction—generally highly related to stress symptoms—provide care which is less good than those with high job satisfaction. For example, Grol (1990) reported that doctors with higher prescription rates and who provided less information for patients showed higher symptoms of frustration and tension. Similarly, other studies link low job satisfaction with lower patient satisfaction, higher no-show rates and lower compliance in patients (Linn et al., 1985; De Matteo et al., 1993).

Mistakes and poor performance, even when they do not result in complaints or litigation, do go on to demoralise doctors in various ways, as these examples (Firth-Cozens and Greenhalgh, 1997) show:

> I missed the diagnosis of pulmonary embolism and treated the patient as a case of severe pneumonia until the day after. The patient's condition deteriorated and only then was the diagnosis put right. I felt guilty and lost confidence.

> Missing a diagnosis of perforated peptic ulcer in a patient—at least she is now well and survived. It made me feel useless at my job though.

It is clear from these findings that the cost to organisations and to patients of psychological distress in all its forms is one that is becoming impossible for managers, the profession and patient organisations to ignore. In this situation it is essential that we isolate its main causes so that appropriate interventions can be made.

CAUSES OF IMPAIRMENT

The finding that depression and stress reduce steadily over the first few years after graduation suggests that rising levels of confidence and competence are likely to have a beneficial effect on one's psychological state (Williams et al., 1997). However, Reuben (1985) found that this did not happen to those in intensive care, and this suggests that job-related factors such as disrupted sleep, high death rates and dealing with distressed relatives may all play a part in producing symptoms. It is important, therefore, to consider both the job-related causes of distress and ones internal to the individual doctor.

Over the past few years much emphasis and energy have been put into the task of reducing the hours of work of doctors in training. Although this was undoubtedly essential, there is only scant evidence that hours were actually related to stress levels, and the reduction in Britain to a maximum of 73 has yet to demonstrate any clear benefits in this regard. In fact, there is some report of dissatisfaction at the reduction in training that might result and the problems in following through patients (see Moss and Paice, Chapter 15 this volume). The evidence on the links between sleep loss and depressed mood is, however, much more compelling (Firth-Cozens, 1993). Although the amount of sleep one has is to some extent dependent upon the hours one works (especially when they exceed 73 per week), the way that sleep is organised also matters: how many interruptions? what is expected of you the next day? and so on. In fact, it may be much more important to create a truly well-functioning team which can organise itself into providing good care for its junior doctors as well as its patients than to continue to attempt simply to reduce hours (Firth-Cozens and Moss, 1998).

Good teams, of course, demand good team leaders, and it is perhaps not surprising that the greatest stressor to the 224 doctors in last assessment, working both in hospitals and general practice, was difficulties with their seniors (Firth-Cozens, 1995). Similarly, Richman et al. (1996) have shown that, for men and for women, workplace abusive relationships such as psychological humiliation and discriminatory treatment, interacting with a vulnerable personality, best predict high alcohol use. It seems likely that senior doctors greatly underestimate the effects, for better or for worse, that they can have on others, and the implications for training in this area are significant (Baldwin et al., 1997b).

Other sources of stress involve the growing expectations of patients, fears about making mistakes, and the increase in litigation and complaints (see Vincent, Chapter 5 this volume). We have seen the consequences of this in North America, and are witnessing its growth in the UK and elsewhere. It makes it especially necessary to organise ways to support doctors who have complaints against them or are suspended, and to reduce the threat of litigation by better communication with patients (Vincent and Bark, 1995; Firth-Cozens, in press).

Beyond these stressors specific to doctors there may be other more general ones which can affect the organisation as a whole: the quality of communication, the clarity of the strategy, the feeling in staff that they are valued, and so on. The finding from Wall et al. (1997) that individual hospitals differ in their levels of stress—from 17% to 33% above threshold on the GHQ and that in larger organisations staff have poorer mental health than in smaller ones—demonstrates clearly just how important good management practice can be. The organisational causes within general practice are described in detail by Howie and Porter (Chapter 12).

Person–job fit

Factors within the workplace meet with those within the individual to produce levels of fit between people and their jobs, which may lead to greater or less stress and satisfaction. Thus the individual may be as important as the workplace in terms of the creation of occupational stress. For example, a number of psychologists over the past few years have emphasised the role of negative affectivity in the creation of life stress (see Payne, Chapter 1); that is, the predisposition in some individuals to experience most aspects of life in a somewhat negative way. However, beyond this general characteristic will be other traits or experiences that affect the person–job fit positively or negatively. In particular, I shall consider the role of early family relationships, career choice, personality and coping style.

It is not only doctors, but health professionals in general who show high levels of stress and depression (Wall *et al.*, 1997), and it has been suggested by psychoanalytic writers that this "helping professions syndrome" (Malan, 1979) may emerge from individuals' needs to make good their early experiences; for example, a depressed parent, early abuse (Elliott and Guy, 1993), parental separation or illness. Certainly, Clark *et al.* (1984) reported that parental depression was predictive of depression in the doctors—a finding borne out further by the AMA–APA Physician Mortality Project, Stage II (APA Council on Scientific Affairs, 1987). Likewise, Paris and Frank (1983) showed that medical students are likely to have had more ill-health in their early families than law students. If these apparently unconscious reasons for choosing medicine lead to unrealistically high expectations and self-criticism, then the uncertainty that is involved in the work of doctors, the lack of support and absence of good "re-parenting" that is common, along with the rising demands and declining gratitude of patients, may well interact to create a potentially depressogenic state involving a sense of failure and self-blame (Firth-Cozens, 1997).

The choice of specialty may also be a feature of earlier individual factors. For example, at the most recent follow-up of my study, psychiatrists were the most stressed (mean of 13.7) and negative about their jobs (2.85), while surgeons were the least (11.3 and 1.67 respectively). While it is possible to see many job-related reasons for this, these differences were just as apparent 10 years earlier when they were students: then students who became psychiatrists were significantly more depressed (6.3) than those who became surgeons. In addition, the psychiatrists as students were the most self-critical group (4.4 compared to 3.6 for surgeons). It may be that some of the psychiatrists had entered the specialty in order to explore their own distress more closely through their patients. Paradoxically, these highly self-critical individuals have chosen a specialty with patients who are much less grateful and more critical than other groups, while it is equally likely the surgeons' patients are quite the opposite in this regard.

Aspects of person–job fit and its effects on stress can also be seen in general practitioners in the study. Raised current high levels of stress and depression were highly predicted by self-criticism and by early sibling rivalry reported as students (0.35, $p<0.001$; Firth-Cozens, 1998). In fact, of the 124 who had become general practitioners, all but 4 had siblings. It may be that they went into this "working family" of the partnership in order to recapture or make good their early family experiences—a strategy which, as in the case of the psychiatrists, has not always been successful.

The importance of early family relationships has been demonstrated in longitudinal studies as well; for example, one looking at the precursors of morbidity and mortality in physicians showed that cold, distant relationships with fathers were predictive of their deaths from suicide and cancer (Thomas and Duszynski, 1974), while Vaillant et al. (1972) found that the physicians were especially likely to have aspects of psychopathology if they had experienced an unhappy childhood. His findings suggested that normal rebellion from parental ties has often been absent, while high levels of altruism may lead to the denial of certain needs that are unlikely to be met in the medical workplace. Similarly, in my study anxious, guilty relationships with mothers was strongly predictive of self-criticism and stress in the first postgraduate year (Firth-Cozens, 1992) and this type of early relationship remains strongly related to their stress scores 10 years later, particularly in women (0.39, $p<0.001$) rather than in men (0.17, $p<0.05$).

A number of personality traits may contribute to stress and depression, but my study has emphasised the role played by high self-criticism in particular (Firth-Cozens, 1997). Regression analyses show that self-criticism as students is a highly significant predictor of depression and stress over the 10 years of the study, especially in men (Brewin and Firth-Cozens, 1997). While high scores predict high symptoms, those reporting poor relationships with seniors, peers and patients have significantly lower self-criticism than others (Firth-Cozens, 1995). It is clear that the healthiest route for doctors and those around them is to take reasonable responsibility for things that go wrong rather than making highly internal or external attributions about them.

An area linked to personality, and also a probable contributor to current stress is the way that individuals cope with the inevitable job-related stressors that face them in medicine. What is clear from my study and others (for example, Koeske *et al.*, 1993; Tyler and Cushway, 1992) is that trying to avoid or dismiss the situation, or deny thoughts about it, are ineffectual ways of coping, as is any form of palliative coping such as alcohol or food bingeing.

Although the lists of potential stressors, both job-related and individual, is long, it is nevertheless true that many of them can be tackled both at the organisational level and throughout undergraduate and postgraduate training, and some suggestions for approaching this follow.

INTERVENTIONS THROUGHOUT TRAINING

The potential problems that individual doctors might find particularly difficult because of their dispositions, coping styles, and so on, might best be addressed during undergraduate and postgraduate training. In fact, some suggest that it should start even earlier, with medical student selection.

The suggestion that medical students might be selected for anything but academic excellence can cause strong reactions and it is certainly true that our evidence for selecting well for any type of occupation is very much in its early stages. Nevertheless, the medical school at the University of Newcastle in New South Wales, Australia, has made a serious attempt over more than two decades to select less narrowly and better, and to follow up their students and compare them to others trained close by but chosen by more traditional means. They have found that their doctors chosen for empathy, problem solving, and a variety of other characteristics agreed to be likely to produce good doctors, actually have greater quality of life and job satisfaction on follow-up after qualification, and no worse academic outcomes than those chosen traditionally (Powis and Rolfe, 1998). At the very least such findings should suggest that we might consider selecting differently and evaluating this systematically. Perhaps more importantly, we may want to consider selecting for entrance into specialties and into consultant grades in much more thorough ways in order to make medicine more akin to other professions, and to maximise the person–job fit.

There are often calls for doctors to have their own occupational health service to deal with problems such as depression and alcohol abuse (Strang *et al.*, 1998), but it may be more important to address doctors' fundamental difficulties in seeking help at all and the apparently casual attitude to self-prescribing (Baldwin *et al.*, 1997b). Part of this reluctance to ask for help is likely to be to do with their splitting off the diseased, disabled and incompetent part of themselves and seeing it as belonging only to patients. Isobel Menzies-Lyth's (1988) work on nurses shows how this was done unconsciously through the strict adherence to uniforms and procedures that separate carer and patient, in order to defend, in a psychological rather than physical sense, the carer's anxieties about death and disease.

In terms of drug use, the profession and its educators need to take an unambivalent stance about excessive use of alcohol, but also encourage young doctors to develop other ways of coping with their stress. Other young professionals are likely to have more time in their first postgraduate years to develop better habits than perhaps they had during student days, but doctors may not have sufficient time or facilities to do this. Other means of tackling stress, such as exercise or social interaction, need to be emphasised both within education and organisationally, and the means to pursue them need to be part of hospital design. Certainly it is important to make access to services easier and better publicised, perhaps also making links with Alcoholics Anonymous which has many medical members both in general groups and in ones consisting just of doctors (Chappel, 1991). The confronting of alcoholic doctors is probably followed more rigorously in the USA than elsewhere (Strang et al., 1998), and these "impaired physician" schemes appear to be relatively successful (Shore, 1987).

In terms of stress management, many of the well-recognised methods,such as relaxation and exercise, are likely to be useful, along with cognitive strategies involving coping skills and changing cognitions in order to confront self-criticism and allow doctors to take reasonable but not excessive responsibility for what goes wrong, and even for what goes right. This is also likely to be an important factor in themes within counselling and psychotherapy, as is the reason for the choice of medicine in the first place, and for the choice of specialty later on. There is an appalling lack of career counselling at any stage of medicine, and prospective candidates for entering particular specialties or even general practice are seldom given the types of psychometric assessments—both skills and psychological state—that we see and expect in other professions.

The provision of other educational inputs, such as handling their own aggression as well as that of colleagues, patients and carers, would undoubtedly be useful. Later in their careers it is important for them to learn to be team leaders, not just by a simple list of skills, but also by their own self-development and understanding.

ORGANISATIONAL RESPONSIBILITIES

Organisations can no longer afford to ignore the elevated stress levels of their staff. The good news is that organisations can make real differences to staff stress, as Wall et al. (1997) have shown in their finding of the wide variation in levels of stress in different hospitals (and see Murphy,

Chapter 11 this volume). Many of these interventions to prevent and lower high stress are actually factors of good management, such as improving communication, changing the culture towards one that can learn from mistakes, and developing good team leaders who can improve their staff's sleep patterns and quality of working life. In addition, policy makers can initiate ways of educating patients about their responsibilities and expectations.

Wall et al.'s (1997) study showed that the better hospitals they surveyed had clear characteristics: greater co-operation, better communication, with more training and discretion for staff. Such factors—similar to those suggested by Vincent et al. (1998) as predictors of better risk management—address the very culture and reflect the general management strategies necessary for the healthy development of any organisation.

Other more specific strategies that organisations can provide to prevent or counteract stress are outlined in the chapters by Murphy (11); Howie and Porter (12); and Wykes and Whittington (17). Secondary interventions also include the provision of stress management courses—which Jones et al. (1988) have shown can also reduce medication errors and claims against the organisation—and counselling services, both internal and external, which may not only reduce absence but also improve job satisfaction and reduce symptoms (Firth-Cozens and Hardy, 1992). It is likely to be especially necessary to direct doctors to such services if there are complaints or litigation against them (see Vincent, Chapter 5).

One of the most useful organisational interventions to improve mental health in the workplace appears to be by developing good teams (Carter and West, Chapter 14): ones which have clear group and individual objectives, which meet regularly and which value the skills of individual members (Guzzo and Shea, 1992). If such teams are multidisciplinary, they can address factors necessary to promote members' well-being in numerous ways: organisational, such as a redistribution of tasks (McKee and Black, 1993); and by being emotionally and practically supportive (Moss and Paice, Chapter 15; Firth-Cozens and Moss, 1998). In particular, one of the most important developments would be that team and organisational culture changes towards the early recognition of stress and any associated poor performance, so that problems can be tackled at once rather than left to develop and increase any impairment.

IN CONCLUSION

This review of stress in doctors has shown that high levels of psychological distress and alcohol abuse exist in the profession, but that we are by now aware of many of the organisational and individual causes of these problems. Moreover, the means exist to address many of these causes, and these should be introduced and evaluated systematically for the sake of doctors' health and to improve the quality of care they are consequently able to give to patients.

REFERENCES

APA Council on Scientific Affairs (1987). Results and implications of the AMA-APA physician mortality project. Stage II. *Journal of the American Medical Association*, **257**, 2949–2953

Baldwin, P.J., Dodd, M. and Wrate, R.W. (1997a). Young doctors' health—I. How do working conditions affect attitudes, health and performance? *Social Science and Medicine*, **45**, 35–40.

Baldwin, P.J., Newton, R.W., Buckley, G., Roberts, M.A. and Dodd, M. (1997b). Senior house officers in medicine: postal survey of training and work experience. *British Medical Journal*, **314**, 740–743.

Bissel, C. and Skorina, J.K. (1987). One hundred alcoholic women in medicine. *Journal of the American Medical Association*, **257**, 2939–2944.

Brewin, C.R. and Firth-Cozens, J. (1997). Dependency and self-criticism as predicting depression in junior doctors. *Journal of Occupational Health*, **2**(3), 242–243.

British Medical Association (1998). Working Group: *The Misuse of Alcohol and Other Drugs by Doctors*. London: British Medical Association.

Brooke, D., Edwards, G. and Taylor, C. (1991). Addiction as an occupational hazard: 144 doctors with drug and alcohol problems. *British Journal of Addiction*, **86**, 1011–1016.

Chappel, J.N. (1991). The use of Alcoholics Anonymous and Narcotics Anonymous by the physician in treating drug and alcohol addiction. In: N.S. Miller (Ed.) *Comprehensive Handbook of Drug and Alcohol Addiction*. New York: Marcel Dekker.

Caplan, R.P. (1994). Stress, anxiety and depression in hospital consultants, general practitioners, and senior health service managers. *British Medical Journal*, **309**, 1261–1263.

Clark, D.C., Salazar-Grueso, E., Grabler, P. and Fawcett, J. (1984). Predictors of depression during the first six months of internship. *American Journal of Psychiatry*, **141**, 1095–1098.

Conrad, S., Hughes, P. and Baldwin, D.C. (1988). Substance use by fourth year students at thirteen medical schools. *Journal of Medical Education*, **63**, 747–58.

Di Matteo, M., Shugars, D.A. and Hays, R.D. (1993). Occupational stress, life stress and mental health among dentists, *Journal of Occupational and Organizational Psychology*, **66**, 153–62.

Elliott, D.M. and Guy, J.D. (1993). Mental health professionals versus non-mental health professionals: childhood trauma and adult functioning. *Professional Psychology: Research and Practice*, **24**(1), 83–90.

Firth-Cozens, J. (1987). Emotional distress in junior house officers. *British Medical Journal*, **295**, 533–536.

Firth-Cozens, J. (1992). The role of early experiences in the perception of organizational stress: fusing clinical and organizational perspectives. *Journal of Occupational and Organizational Psychology*, **65**, 61–75.

Firth-Cozens, J. (1993). Stress, psychological problems, and clinical performance. In C. Vincent, M. Ennis and R.M.J. Audley (Eds) *Medical Accidents*. Oxford: Oxford University Press.

Firth-Cozens, J. (1995). Sources of stress in junior doctors and general practitioners. *Yorkshire Medicine*, **7**, 10–13.

Firth-Cozens, J. (1997). Depression in doctors. In C. Katona and M.M. Robertson (Eds) *Depression and Physical Illness*. Chichester: Wiley.

Firth-Cozens, J. (1998). Individual and organisational predictors of depression in general practitioners. *British Journal of General Practice*, **48**, 1647–1651.

Firth-Cozens, J. (in press). Interventions to improve physician wellbeing and patient care, *Social Science and Medicine*.

Firth-Cozens, J. and Greenhalgh, J. (1997). Doctors' perceptions of the links between stress and lowered clinical care. *Social Science and Medicine*, **44**(7), 1017–1022.

Firth-Cozens, J. and Hardy, G. (1992). Occupational stress, clinical treatment and changes in job perceptions, *Journal of Occupational and Organizational Psychology*, **65**, 81–88.

Firth-Cozens, J. and Moss, F. (1998). Hours, sleep, teamwork and stress. *British Medical Journal*, **317**, 1335–1336.

Flaherty, J.A. and Richman, J.A. (1993). Substance use and addiction among medical students, residents and physicians. *Recent Advances in Addictive Disorders*, **16**(1), 189–97.

Goldberg, D. (1978). *Manual of the General Heatlh Questionniare*. Windsor: NFER.

Grol, R. (1990). National standard setting for quality of care in general practice: attitudes of general practitioners and responses to a set of standards. *British Journal of General Practice*, **40**, 361–364.

Gross, E.B. (1997). Gender differences in physician stress: Why the discrepant findings? *Women and Health*, **26**, 1–14.

Guzzo, R.A. and Shea, G.P. (1992). Group performance and intergroup relations. In M.D. Dunnette and L.M. Hough, (Eds) *Handbook of Industrial and Organisational Psychology* (pp. 269–313). Palo Alto, CA: Consulting Psychologists Press.

Harrison, D. and Chick, J. (1994). Trends in alcoholism among male doctors in Scotland. *Addiction*, **89**, 1613–1617.

Jones, J.W., Barge, B.N., Steffy, B.D., Fay, L.M., Junz, L.K. and Wvebeker, L.J. (1988). Stress and medical malpractice: organisational risk assessment and intervention. *Journal of Applied Psychology*, **4**, 727–735.

Khantzian, E.J. and Mack, J.E. (1994). How AA works and why it's important for clinicians to understand. *Journal of Substance Abuse Treatment*, **11**, 77–92.

Koeske, G.F., Kirk, S.A. and Koeske, R.D. (1993). Coping with job stress: Which strategies work best? *Journal of Occupational and Organizational Psychology*, **66**, 319–335.

Linn, L.S., Brook, R.H., Clark, V.A. and Ross Davies, A. (1985). Physician and patient satisfaction as factors related to the organization of internal medicine group practices. *Medical Care*, **23**, 1171–1178.

Malan, D.H. (1979). *Individual Psychotherapy and the Science of Psycho-dynamics*. London: Butterworths.

Menzies-Lyth, I. (1988). *Containing Anxiety in Institutions*. London: Free Associations Press.

McKee, M. and Black, N. (1992). Does the current use of junior doctors in the United Kingdom affect the quality of medical care? *Social Science and Medicine,* **34**, 549–558.

McKee, M. and Black, N. (1993). Junior doctors' work at night: What is done and how much is appropriate? *Journal of Public Health Medicine,* **15**, 16–24.

Orton, D.I. and Gruzelier, J.H. (1989). Adverse changes in mood and cognitive performance of house officers after night duty. *British Medical Journal,* **298**, 21–23.

Paris, J. and Frank, H. (1983). Psychological determinants of a medical career. *Canadian Journal of Psychiatry,* **28**, 354–357.

Powis, D.A. and Rolfe, I. (1998). Selection and performance of medical students at Newcastle, New South Wales. *Education for Health,* **11**, 15–23.

Pullen, D., Lonie, C.E, Lyle, D.M., Cam, D.E. and Doughty, M.V. (1995). The medical care of doctors. *Medical Journal of Australia,* **162**, 481–484.

Reuben, D.B. (1985). Depressive symptoms in medical house officers: effects of level of training and work rotation. *Archives of International Medicine,* **145**, 286–288

Richman, J.A., Flaherty, J.A. and Rospenda, K.M. (1996). Perceived workplace harassment experiences and problem drinking among physicians: broadening the stress/alienation paradigm. *Addiction,* **91**(3), 391–403.

Rucinski, J. and Cybulska, E. (1985). Mentally ill doctors. *British Journal of Hospital Medicine,* **33**, 90–94

Sclare, B. (1979). Alcoholism in doctors. *British Journal of Alcohol and Alcoholism,* **14**, 181–196.

Shore, J.H. (1987). The Oregon experience with impaired physicians on probation: an 8-year follow-up. *Journal of the American Medical Association,* **257**, 2931–2934.

Sonnetag, S. (1996). Work group factors and individual well-being. In M.A. West (Ed.) *Handbook of Work Group Psychology.* Chichester: Wiley.

Strang, J., Wilks, M., Wells, B. and Marshall, J. (1998). Missed problems and missed opportunities for addicted doctors. *British Medical Journal,* **316**, 405–406.

Thomas, C.B. and Duszynski, K.R. (1974). Closeness to parents and the family constellation in a prospective study of five disease states: suicide, mental illness, malignant tumour, hypertension and coronary heart disease. *Johns Hopkins Medical Journal,* **134**, 251–270.

Tyler, P. and Cushway, D. (1992). Stress, coping and mental wellbeing in hospital nurses. *Stress Medicine,* **8**, 91–98.

Vaillant, G.E., Sobowale, N. and McArthur, C. (1972). Some psychological vulnerabilities of physicians. *New England School of Medicine,* **287**, 372–375.

Vincent, C.A. and Bark, P. (1995). Accident investigation:discovering why things go wrong. In Vincent, C.A. (Ed.) *Clinical Risk Management* (pp. 391–410). London: BMJ Publications.

Vincent, C.A., Taylor-Adams, S. and Stanhope, N. (1998). Framework for analysing risk and safety in clinical medicine. *British Medical Journal,* 316, 1154–1157.

Wall, T.D., Bolden, R.I., Borril, C.S., Carter, A.J., Golya, D.A., Hardy, G.E., Haynes, C.E., Rick, J.E., Shapiro, D. and West, M. (1997). Minor psychiatric disorder in NHS trust staff: occupational and gender differences. *British Journal of Psychiatry,* **171**, 519–523.

Williams, S., Dale, J., Glucksman, E. and Wellesley, A. (1997). Senior house officers' work related stressors, psychological distress, and confidence in performing clinical tasks in accident and emergency: a questionnaire study. *British Medical Journal,* **314**, 713–718.

7

NURSING

Pamela J. Baldwin

INTRODUCTION

There has been concern for a long time about the physical and mental health of nurses. They are at high risk of physical illness, especially low back pain, through exposure to hazardous environments (Smedley *et al.*, 1997), and they are vulnerable to mental illness (Tyler and Cushway, 1992) and suicide (Charlton, 1995). This concern over health has extended to nurses in training, where the source of stress is thought to come from both adjustment to clinical contact with patients and the academic pressures (e.g. Rhead, 1995).

One of the difficulties in examining nurses' health and welfare is the diversity of their roles within the health services. Cross-sectional studies may sample nurses in any variety of settings, from close teamwork for emergency care in hospital to the individual nurse practising long-term palliative care in the community. In general, the main principles of occupational stress emerge repeatedly: the importance of job control; a manageable workload; good communication; and social support. How these factors apply to nurses may vary over time and setting. In practice it is important to identify the concrete variables: What constitutes a high workload or adequate support from other staff? The importance of individual factors also needs further research. It is known that there are variations in how working conditions interact with individual personality and coping style (e.g, Dewe, 1989) but such relationships are complex and comparatively unexplored. A second major methodological problem is that the effects of stress are measured in many different ways: job

Stress in Health Professionals. Edited by Jenny Firth-Cozens and Roy L. Payne
© 1999 John Wiley & Sons Ltd

satisfaction; mental health; sickness-absence; tension and tiredness, depression, "burnout"; or post-traumatic stress disorder. This chapter aims to tease apart some of the diversity of current findings before pooling the common threads and identifying what might be acted upon to improve working conditions.

STRESS IN NURSES IN TRAINING

For students, there are the two aspects of training with the potential to be stressful: in common with qualified nurses, there are the clinical pressures of working with patients who are vulnerable and needy; and alongside this, the strain of completing an academic course. In common with other students, they have the problems of leaving home, financial constraints, examinations and the constant scrutiny of academic and clinical staff. West and Rushton (1986) found that among nurses in training, scores on the General Health Questionnaire increased over time, indicating that the psychological symptoms worsened as nurses progressed through training. A similar finding is described by Brunt (1984) for student nurses in an Accident and Emergency setting. Rather than nurses settling down over the course of training, they appear to become more distressed.

Student midwives have reported stress as coming from a variety of factors (Cavanagh and Snape, 1997). Most pronounced for this particular sample was the risk of unemployment after completing the course. This concern is likely to vary over time and across countries, and even within countries, but indicates the importance of monitoring stress in the context of time and place. Another major source of stress was the academic load and its organisation, for which there were significant differences between those students on the shortened pre-registration course and those on the full pre-registration course. The next major source of stress was the work/home interface.

In the UK, particular interest has been generated by a major change in the curriculum for nurses in training. There has been a move away from the apprentice model of nurse training, where nurses had early clinical experience and were considered part of the workforce throughout training. The new model, named Project 2000 (P2000), sees nurses as scientist-practitioners, with a depth of knowledge and theory that is applied to the clinical setting. They are students, rather than employees, and their status is supernumerary on the wards. This was intended as a way of removing clinical pressure while they learned and reflected upon their practice. Such a change has made people curious to know not only whether this training is more appropriate to current nursing practice, but also whether it is more or less stressful than the former style.

Rhead (1995) compared second-year P2000 students with RGN nurses in their third year, whose training had been apprenticeship-style on the wards and found that the latter group reported less stress although, somewhat surprisingly, the stress reported was greater for practical rather than academic work. P2000 students reported more stress for both components. This comparison suggests that courses exert different strains, but since the participants of the study were from different stages within each course, there are limitations in the conclusions. Specific difficulties have been reported with the initiation of P2000 training. In a series of detailed case studies in colleges of training in Scotland, May *et al.* (1997) examined the early intakes for the new course and indicated strengths and weaknesses of the innovation, as well as the directions for future development of the curriculum. Similar points were outlined by Jowett (1995). There has been concern about the lack of integration between course aims, methods and philosophy and clinical staff on the placements, as well as the need for earlier clinical skills teaching (Hamill, 1995). On the other hand, the depth, breadth and relevance of the course content has been praised by students (Parker and Carlisle, 1996). The course is in continuing evolution and it is not yet clear to what extent these early teething troubles have been remedied.

The type of nursing experienced during training has also been shown to be associated with differences. Parkes (1980) compared student nurses on medical and surgical wards and found reduced satisfaction and higher anxiety and depression for those in medicine. It was hypothesised that the exposure to chronic illness among medical patients was more distressing than caring for the short-stay surgical patients.

Training is not always associated with increased distress. There is some evidence from USA that for more mature students, who return to further academic training in advanced skills, this education offers a buffer against burnout, particularly when it is associated with peer and family social support (Dick and Anderson, 1993). Training in this situation might offer new hope, and new possibilities for practice that combat the disengagement that is characteristic of burnout in the caring professions.

When comparing nurses in training, the picture is quite complex and reinforces an interaction model looking at the type and stage of training, the clinical setting and the nature of the individuals entering training. In the next section, the factors influencing qualified nurses are examined.

QUALIFIED NURSES

As nurses work in a wide variety of settings and roles, it is important to extract the various comparisons that have been made and to be aware of the different aspects of the working environment and the measures of stress that have been used. Nursing remains a predominantly female profession, therefore most of the results reported will be for women, unless otherwise specified.

Different settings

Early studies concentrated on areas of intensive care (e.g. special care baby units, coronary care units) but it seems that these are not necessarily more stressful than other areas (Gentry and Parkes, 1982). As indicated above, it is likely that buffering effects, such as staff cohesion, teamwork and a heightened awareness of the demanding nature of the work, mediate between the demands of critical care and the individual nurse. For example, Hare et al. (1988) discovered that institutions showing an interest in monitoring levels of burnout were those whose staff reported highest levels of job satisfaction and lowest levels of burnout. Thus an institution that is aware of the risks is likely to be a healthier workplace than one that does not wish to address the problem.

A growing area of concern is the risk of violence to which nurses are exposed. In particular medical settings there is an increasing risk of physical assault upon nurses, e.g. in Accident and Emergency and psychiatric inpatient units. Whittington and Wykes (1992) carried out a detailed study of incidents in a psychiatric hospital. Although most of these resulted in no detectable physical injury, and the majority of staff showed levels of anxiety afterwards that were within the normal range, some staff reacted with symptoms of post-traumatic stress disorder (PTSD). In these incidents, a nurse may suffer typical symptoms of PTSD: anxiety and insomnia, flashbacks, heightened vigilance, etc., long after the incident. Interestingly, informal support was often given to the victim immediately after the incident, but not thereafter, despite the fact that in this study, the distress could last several weeks. In the case of PTSD, it is known that this can develop months later, or persist for years. Evidence from the USA suggests that male nurses may be more at risk of such assault, since they are often called to deal with violent incidents before female staff (Hiscott and Connop, 1989).

Qualified nurses compared with unqualified nurses and those in training

Wall et al. (1997) found that senior, managerial nursing staff reported more distress than other nursing staff, but this latter group did not include student nurses. A different cross-sectional survey of one health board area revealed that unqualified nurses had significantly less stress than qualified nurses, whereas students had more (Jones, 1994). This underlines the importance of separating out the different variables of nursing experience and qualification when looking at stress.

SUMMARY OF EXISTING LITERATURE

Overwhelmingly, studies of stress among nurses are cross-sectional in design. In general, the main stressors which appear frequently are high workload, lack of staff support, contact with critically ill patients, and the emotional demands of patients and relatives (e.g. Gray-Toft and Anderson, 1985; Dewe, 1987; Guppy and Gutteridge, 1991). The emphasis has tended to be on environmental models of stress, i.e. the nature of the job, rather than interaction between the individual and the environment (Wheeler and Riding, 1994).

Yet the relationships between the context, the stage of career, and individual style are complicated. Longitudinal studies are needed to tease out the factors. It seems likely that preventative strategies for problems in the nursing career have to be tailor-made for the nurse and the setting. In the next section new evidence will be presented to address some of the questions prompted by findings so far. These questions concern what might be done to alleviate the stress among nurses.

A LONGITUDINAL STUDY OF NURSES

Data presented here come from a longitudinal study undertaken by the author and colleagues (Baldwin *et al.*, 1998). The study extended over four years.

Subjects and methods

Four class cohorts were recruited. Two UK universities were chosen as the study sites. The first-year P2000 classes and the leaving classes of the old style of training were recruited to take part at each site. Compliance rates for personal interview in the first year of the study were 67% for leavers and 74% for P2000 students. Compliance rates among consenters for two annual postal follow-ups and a final interview ranged from 70 to 94% for each of the cohorts. The measures used were extensive, but those reported here are the GHQ-28 (Goldberg and Hillier, 1979) as well as self-reported sickness-absence and days at work but unfit for duty. The GHQ-28 is a screening device for psychological symptoms. This version has the benefit of separate subscales: somatic symptoms, anxiety and insomnia, social dysfunction and severe depression. In addition, an

Attitudes to Work questionnaire (Firth-Cozens, 1992) was adapted for application to the cohorts of leaving nurses. This is a 25-item scale covering various aspects of their job along dimensions which are established as influential in most working environments. This scale was collapsed down into factors, which changed in number and associated variance from year to year during the follow-up.

For the leaving nurses, after they had left college and were working in nursing, the first factor to emerge remained the same every year: it had an eigenvalue of 4.8 or greater and accounted for most of the variance (greater than 20%) each year. This factor is termed "Senior support and communication", with highest loadings for statements such as "I have attention paid to suggestions that I make", "Senior staff let me know how well I am doing", and "I can discuss work problems with senior staff", etc. The factor emerging second varied from year to year, and accounted for 11% of the variance or less.

For the P2000 classes the picture was different. Their context was that of a learner, and social support at work was not as important as education. For them, there was a purpose-designed questionnaire which covered academic tasks as well as clinical training. The simple 5-point scales reported here were concerned with the amount that the students were learning on placement, and the ease with which difficulties on placement could be resolved.

Results will be discussed with reference to the three levels of possible intervention to alleviate stress in nursing.

Primary prevention

Primary prevention of stress in nursing may start in selecting personnel with resistance or "hardiness", or with structuring a job and its climate in such a way as to ameliorate the effects of pressure on the job.

Selection

Would it be possible to identify nursing applicants who were likely to be vulnerable to stress and advise them against entering the profession? To test this, one would need to know which factors among first-year students were predictive of subsequent mental health problems or drop-out from the profession. Using the data from the longitudinal study of P2000 students, it is possible to look at such factors annually. Between the first and second year of their three-year course, a total of 16 of the 212 participating P2000 students had left nurse training. All were contacted and asked to fill in a brief questionnaire on their reasons for leaving. Ten people responded: the majority said that they had left due to personal circumstances. Data from the first year on all 16 student nurses were compared with those still in training: they did not differ significantly in terms of mental or physical health, days at work but unfit, or days off sick.

It seems that dropping out from training during the first year is unlikely to be related to mental instability but rather a collection of miscellaneous personal circumstances that could not have been foreseen. The same data were examined at the end of the three-year training course. The nurses were divided into three groups: those known to have left at some point before the end of the course; those whose qualification was delayed (as a result of illness or time out for any reason); and those who qualified within the three years. Looking back at these students' GHQ-28 symptoms in first year, those who finished on time had the fewest psychological symptoms in first year (lowest GHQ-28 score) followed by those finishing late, then those who dropped out. However, these differences were not statistically significant (Kruskal-Wallis ANOVA, $\chi^2 = 3.35$. Results are given in Table 7.1.

It appears, looking at P2000 students entering training, that there is unlikely to be a reliable psychological assessment that would identify the successful qualifiers from the rest.

Table 7.1: First year scores as students on the GHQ-28

Nursing group	N	Mean GHQ-28 score in first year	Range
Those qualifying on time	149	16.8	1–52
Those qualifying late	21	17.5	5–56
Those who left before qualifying	42	19.7	6–41
Total	212	17.5	1–56

Secondary intervention

Staff support

Looking at the leaving classes in our study, we can examine their state of health over three years of work as a qualified nurse. "Senior support" was negatively correlated with GHQ-28 total scores in each year ($r = -0.27$, $r = -0.30$ and $r = -0.22$, $p < 0.05$), indicating that higher levels of support and communication with senior staff were significantly associated with fewer psychological symptoms in every year of the follow-up.

Initiating support for staff

If senior support is not occurring spontaneously, then interventions focusing on supervision might facilitate the process. Marriott (1991) outlines the accumulated evidence for this. The amount of time that a trainer spends with a trainee appears to be critical: it is the approachability and availability of the trainer that matters. Although this can be difficult to ensure with the heavy demands on all nursing staff, these "player managers" have been shown to be extremely important for effective learning and support in a variety of medical training settings (Wilson et al., 1996).

Staff support systems have been employed in many settings but there is very little data on the evaluation of the efficacy of such groups. In a qualitative account of a staff support system, Jenkins and Stevenson (1991) describe the establishment of a peer support group with explicit ground rules. It serves to enable staff to discuss their responses to clinical and managerial events, to show appreciation of one another's strengths and to aid communication about the organisation of work and resources. There has been no formal evaluation of this structure, but once established, this model "spawned" others throughout the district.

There are difficulties in carrying out research into the effectiveness of interventions designed to increase staff support. Measurement of the subtle changes in attitude and behaviour are problematic; staff change shifts; are often only temporarily in post; and it is difficult to design an experimental intervention with either an appropriate control group or with a stable condition where the initiation of a staff support group is the only change at work that takes place.

Teamwork

Teams are one method of formalising a support system. The concept of teamwork implies that workers share responsibility and decision making, carrying out their duties with reference to the strengths and needs of other workers. A review of this aspect appears in Chapter 14. Good teams are characterised by effective communication, with clear and complementary roles for members of the team. In nursing, an intervention study attempted to reduce stress among nurses by creating small teams of four nursing and administrative staff who looked after a limited number of 10 to 12 patients (Murphy et al., 1994). Each member of the team had a different role and grade, but together they provided the total care for all their patients. This reorganisation into teams resulted in greater cooperation and reduced stress. Within nursing, however, attention has focused on an even smaller unit of staff. In place of teamworking, there has been the development of "primary" nursing, where each qualified nurse has the main responsibility for an even smaller number of patients. Where primary nursing has been compared with team nursing, or functional nursing (a task-based division of labour) it has been shown to be associated with positive outcomes: these include not only greater autonomy and less work pressure for both senior grades and unqualified nurses, but greater peer cohesion and supervisor support (Thomas, 1992). In a review of this issue, Gardner (1991) concludes that, overall, primary nursing results in higher quality of care and reduced turnover of nursing staff, particularly qualified staff. These studies indicate that it is possible to change the organisational structure of the job to improve the quality of nursing as well as the pressure of the job.

Tertiary intervention

When nurses become seriously distressed, for whatever reason, they have access not only to their own family doctor, but to an occupational health service. Comparatively little is known of the usage of this service, but in a UK survey Mayberry et al. (1986) identified that the majority of staff were aware of the service, wanted it, and had used it. The survey identified that nurses wanted certain services significantly more than other professional groups. Among these services was "counselling".

In our own longitudinal study, the leaving cohort of nurses was asked to report their beliefs about the Occupational Health Service both at the final year in training and after three years as qualified employees. They were given three different conditions and asked to say whether they believed that the Occupational Health Physician would have a role at any of the three different listed stages. Results are shown in Table 7.2.

For all three conditions their perceptions of the Occupational Health Physician's role increased over time. After they had worked for three

Table 7.2: Leaving nurses' beliefs during training and in clinical practice about the role of an Occupational Health Physician at three stages of three different conditions

	Assessment of the condition (%)	Arranging treatment (%)	Assessing fitness for work (%)
Muscular-skeletal disorder:	82	59	75
Final year at College (N=147)	87	62	78
After 3 years service (N=118)			
Depression:	48	32	42
Final year at College (N=147)	63	50	59
After 3 years service (N=118)			
Alcohol/substance dependency:	61	46	56
Final year at College (N=147)	73	63	62
After 3 years service (N=118)			

years, the majority saw that both physical and mental health were within the remit of the service, although there remain large proportions who do not think it appropriate to consult for any of the defined conditions. More worrying is the finding that, during their last year at college, 59% of the classes thought that the service was entirely confidential and this changed negligibly after they had worked for three years. This is despite the fact that, in the UK, the Faculty of Occupational Medicine (1993) has issued clear guidelines on the confidentiality of information, which may be disclosed only in explicitly listed circumstances.

SUMMARY

Stress in nursing may come from many different sources depending on the setting, the organisation of the nursing role and the response of the individual to the circumstances. There will be no single remedy for the problem, but rather every individual needs to be considered in the light of the context in which he or she works. Providing Occupational Health Services, or other therapeutic agencies with easy access for nurses, is essential but this is tertiary intervention: it is acting after the damage has been done. Primary prevention, in terms of selecting out people who are less able to cope with stress, is unlikely to be reliable. Major attention needs to be drawn to the secondary level. The first step is for the institution to recognise the risk of stress and burnout. The next step is to examine the structural and managerial aspects of nursing that contribute to the development of stress in nurses. Team nursing appears to provide a healthier working environment than functional nursing. Evidence suggests that primary nursing, in effect a very small team, offers staff the best conditions for minimising stress: high levels of control, a clear role, the opportunity to make decisions and structured staff support.

There is much common ground in the influential factors for nurses' health at work, but the literature also demonstrates the diversity of findings. It calls for site-specific interventions which begin with a detailed analysis of the situation, before recommending the way forward. The interest and the challenge lies in combining the universal principles with the characteristics that are unique to each nurse in each nursing role.

ACKNOWLEDGEMENTS

Thanks are due to all nurses who took part in the longitudinal study reported here, and to the Chief Scientist's Office, Scottish Office, for supporting the project.

REFERENCES

Baldwin, P.J., Dodd, M. and Wrate, R.M. (1998). *Young Nurses: Work, Health and Welfare*. Report for the Chief Scientist's Office, Scottish Office, UK.

Brunt, C. (1984). Stress and student nurses in A&E: assessing anxiety levels. *Nursing Times*, **80**, 37–38.

Cavanagh, S.J. and Snape, J. (1997). Educational sources of stress in midwifery students. *Nurse Education Today*, **17**, 128–134.

Charlton, J. (1995). Trends and patterns in suicide in England and Wales. *International Journal of Epidemiology*, **24**, S45-S52.

Dewe, P.J. (1987). Identifying the causes of nurses' stress: a survey of New Zealand nurses. *Work and Stress*, **1**, 15–24.

Dewe, P.J. (1989). Stressor frequency, tension, tiredness and coping: some measurement issues and a comparison across nursing groups. *Journal of Advanced Nursing*, **14**, 308–320.

Dick, M. and Anderson, S.E. (1993) Job burnout in RN-to-BSN students: relationships to life stress, time commitments, and support for returning to school. *Journal of Continuing Education in Nursing*, **24**, 105–109.

Faculty of Occupational Medicine (1993). *Guidance on Ethics for Occupational Physicians. Fourth Edition.*

Firth-Cozens, J. (1992). The role of early family experiences in the perception of organisational stress: fusing clinical and organisational perspectives. *Journal of Occupational and Organizational Psychology*, **65**, 61–75.

Gardner , K. (1991) A summary of findings of a five-year comparison study of primary and team nursing. *Nursing Research*, **40**(2), 113–117.

Gentry, W.D. and Parkes, K.R. (1982). Psychological stress in intensive care unit and non-intensive care unit nursing: a review of the past decade. *Heart and Lung: Journal of Critical Care*, **11**, 43–47.

Goldberg, D.P. and Hillier, V.F. (1979). A scaled version of the General Health Questionnaire. *Psychological Medicine*, **9**, 139–145.

Gray-Toft, P.A. and Anderson, J.G. (1985). Organizational stress in the hospital: development of a model for diagnosis and prediction. *Health Services Research*, **19**, 753–774.

Guppy, A. and Gutteridge, T. (1991). Job satisfaction and occupational stress in UK general hospital nursing staff. *Work and Stress*, **5**, 315–323.

Hamill, C. (1995). The phenomenon of stress as perceived by Project 2000 student nurses: a case study. *Journal of Advanced Nursing*, **21**, 528–536.

Hare, J., Pratt, C.C. and Andrews, D. (1988). Predictors of burnout in professional and paraprofessional nurses working in hospitals and nursing homes. *International Journal of Nursing Studies*, **25**, 105–115.

Hiscott, R.D. and Connop, P.J. (1989). Job stress and occupational burnout: gender differences among mental health professionals. *Sociology and Social Research*, **74**, 10–15.

Jenkins, E. and Stevenson, I. (1991). A strategy for managing change and stress: developing staff support groups. *Professional Nurse*, **6**, 579–581.

Jones, L. (1994). *The Lothian Health Healthy Workplace Strategy: the "Health at Work" Survey*. Final Report, Scottish Health Feedback, Leamington Terrace, Edinburgh, UK.

Jowett, S. (1995). Nurse education in the 1900s: the implementation of the pre-registration Diploma course (Project 2000). *Nurse Education Today*, **15**, 39–43.

Marriott, A. (1991). The support, supervision and instruction of nurse learners in clinical areas: a literature review. *Nurse Education Today*, **12**, 261–269.

May, N., Veitch, L., McIntosh, J.B. and Alexander, M.F. (1997). *Preparation for practice: evaluation of Nurse and Midwife Education in Scotland. Final Report*, Glasgow: Caledonian University.

Mayberry, J.F., Foulis, W. and Street, C.M. (1986). The role of occupational health units in hospital: an assessment by employees. *Social Science and Medicine*, **23**, 469–470.

Murphy, R., Pearlman, F., Rea, C. and Papazian-Boyce, L. (1994). Work redesign: a return to the basics. *Nursing Management*, **25**, 37–39.

Parker, T.J. and Carlisle, C. (1996). Project 2000 students' perceptions of their training. *Journal of Advanced Nursing*, **24**, 771–778.

Parkes, K.R. (1980). Occupational stress among student nurses—1. A comparison of medical and surgical wards. *Nursing Times*, **76**, 117.

Rhead, M.M. (1995). Stress among student nurses: is it practical or academic? *Journal of Clinical Nursing*, **4**, 369–376.

Riding, R.J. and Wheeler, H.H. (1995). Occupational stress and cognitive style in nurses: 1. *British Journal of Nursing*, **4**, 103–106.

Smedley, J., Egger, P., Cooper, C. and Coggon, D. (1997). Prospective cohort study of predictors of incident low back pain in nurses. *British Medical Journal*, **314**, 1225–1228.

Thomas, L.H. (1992). Qualified nurse and nursing auxiliary perceptions of their work environment in primary, team and functional nursing wards. *Journal of Advanced Nursing*, **17**, 373–382.

Tyler, P. and Cushway, D. (1992). Stress, coping and mental well-being in hospital nurses. *Stress Medicine*, **8**, 91–98.

Wall, T.D., Bolden, R.I., Borrill, C.S., Carter, A.J., Golya, D.A., Hardy, G.E., Haynes, C.E., Rick, J.E., Shapiro, D.A. and West, M.A. (1997). Minor psychiatric disorder in NHS trust staff: occupational and gender differences. *British Journal of Psychiatry*, **171**, 519–523.

West, M. and Rushton, R. (1986). The drop-out factor. *Nursing Times*, Dec. 31, **52**, 29–31.

Wheeler, H. and Riding, R. (1994). Occupational stress in general nurses and midwives. *British Journal of Nursing*, **3**, 527–534.

Whittington, R. and Wykes, T. (1992). Staff strain and social support in a psychiatric hospital following assault by a patient. *Journal of Advanced Nursing*, **17**, 480–486.

Wilson, V. Finnigan, J., Pittie, A. and McFall, E. (1996). *Encouraging learning: Lessons from Scottish Health Organisations*. Research Report from the Scottish Council for Research in Education, Edinburgh EH8 8JR.

8

HEALTH SERVICE
MANAGERS

Carol Borrill and Clare Haynes

INTRODUCTION

Managers have a critical role in organisations, and are central to organisational effectiveness (Salaman, 1995). The cost to organisations if managers do not function effectively in their role is therefore considerable (Cooper and Melhuish, 1984). Explanations and causes of ineffective management are many and varied, but one of the most plausible and proved reasons is that they are suffering from stress.

This chapter focuses on the nature and likely causes of work and organisational stress for managers in the health sector, and outlines a range of approaches for reducing stress among these managers.

MANAGERS IN HEALTH CARE ORGANISATIONS

There is considerable variation in the activities, functions and responsibilities of managers in health care organisations, ranging from executive directors, responsible for strategic and operational decisions which shape the organisation's future, through to first line managers, such as team leaders and ward managers, who work alongside clinical staff delivering health care services to the public. Increasingly clinicians are involved in management so there are a growing number of managers from across all the professional groups who are both actively involved in the delivery of

Stress in Health Professionals. Edited by Jenny Firth-Cozens and Roy L. Payne
© 1999 John Wiley & Sons Ltd

care, and responsible for management decisions about this care, including the allocation and use of resources.

CAUSES OF STRESS AMONG MANAGERS

There is a substantial body of research evidence on the sources of work-related stress for managers (see Cooper and Marshall, 1978; Cooper and Melhuish, 1984), but there is little research evidence about the prevalence and causes of stress among health care managers. The general work and organisational sources of stress have been discussed in Chapter 1. However, Burke (1988) identified four additional sources of stress of specific relevance to managers. First, during mergers and acquisitions work stressors are heightened, including uncertainty and threat (Gill and Foulder, 1978), loss of personal and organisational identities and feelings of conflict. Second, organisational retrenchment and decline, when organisations become "meaner and leaner" (Hirschorn, 1983), subjects staff to various sources of stress (Jick, 1983), including role confusion, job insecurity, work overload, career plateauing and poor incentives. Third, a more recent change in organisations has been the overturn of traditionally secure managerial and professional jobs into insecure ones (Hunt, 1986). This has resulted in job future ambiguity and insecurity, which is as detrimental to health as job loss itself. Finally, occupational locking-in arises among managers who have almost no opportunity to move from their present job, and is found to relate to greater negative states and less life satisfaction (Wolpin and Burke, 1986).

Managers are exposed to a wide range of organisational and work-related sources of stress, and a number of studies suggest that this may result in managers experiencing levels of stress which are higher than other occupational groups. Turnage and Spielberger (1991) found that managers reported experiencing job pressures, such as lack of support, more often than professionals/engineers, but attributed less stress intensity to these pressures. Mullarkey et al. (1998) report considerable variations in the prevalence of stress (using the GHQ-12; Goldberg, 1972) across a wide range of occupational groups, with the highest rate (31%), being among managers.

HEALTH CARE MANAGERS

The prevalence of stress: comparisons between private sector and public sector managers

The general consensus is that the role of managers is demanding and they are exposed to a wide range of work and organisational sources of stress. Evidence supporting this conclusion is drawn from managers working in a wide range of sectors, suggesting that these factors associated with stress are generic. However, discussion of the differences between managers working in public and private sector organisations suggests that the former may be exposed to additional work role and organisational stressors. There is some evidence to support this contention.

First, comparisons between the prevalence of stress among managers in the NHS (Borrill *et al.*, 1998), managers in the British Household Panel Survey (BHPS) (1997), and managers in manufacturing (West *et al.*, 1995) show the prevalence of stress to be higher among health care managers.

Table 8.1 shows that the prevalence of stress among NHS managers is substantially and significantly higher than for managers in the BHPS and manufacturing.

Second, other research studies involving health care managers, have reported high levels of stress. For example, Caplan (1994), using the GHQ-12, reported a prevalence rate of 31% among NHS managers, and Litwinenko and Cooper (1995), using the Occupational Stress Indicator (OSI) (Cooper *et al.*, 1988), reported high levels of emotional ill-health among senior health care managers.

Table 8.1:   Comparison of stress among NHS and non-NHS managers

Type of manager	Number	% Stress*
NHS managers	934	32.8
BHPS managers	809	21.3
Manufacturing managers	1126	23.0

* Stress was measured in all above studies using the GHQ-12 (Goldberg, 1972), (3/4 caseness cut-off)

The prevalence of stress: comparisons between managers and other occupational groups in health care

There is conflicting evidence as to whether the prevalence of stress among health service managers is higher than in other occupational groups working in health care organisations. Caplan (1994) found no differences in the prevalence of stress among managers, consultants and general practitioners. Litwinenko and Cooper (1995), however, reported that emotional ill-health was poorer among senior managers in comparison with other occupational groups.

A large-scale longitudinal study of NHS employees, carried out in 17 public health care provider units (NHS Trusts) (Borrill *et al.*, 1998; Wall *et al.*, 1997) has consistently shown that the prevalence of stress is higher among managers than staff in other occupational groups (i.e. nurses, doctors, professions allied to medicine, professional and technical staff, ancillary staff, administrative staff). These are managers who work in an exclusively managerial role, or an administrative role with supervisory responsibility, but do not have any clinical responsibilities. The prevalence of stress was measured, using the GHQ-12, at two time points, with two years between surveys. The proportion of managers who reported experiencing stress at Time 2 was 32.8%, not substantially different from that reported two years previously, 33.4%. At both time points this level was significantly higher than among the other NHS occupational groups. The prevalence of stress across the main occupational groups at Time 2 is shown in Table 8.2.

Table 8.2:   Comparison of the prevalence of stress among the major occupational groups in the NHS

Occupational group	Number	% Stress*
Managers	994	32.8
Nurses	4236	27.6
Professions allied to medicine	1502	26.8
Professional and technical staff	730	25.8
Doctors	1235	24.6
Administrative staff	1801	23.5
Ancillary staff	567	23.1

* Stress was measured using the GHQ-12 (Goldberg, 1972)

Work-related factors associated with stress among health care managers

Using self-report measures of work role factors (e.g. work demands, role conflict, social support), the study described above identified sources of stress experienced by staff working in NHS trusts. The results from the Time 2 data collection are reported here, and are illustrated with quotes from the health care managers. The main work-related factors associated with stress for managers were:

- *Work demand*   The extent to which individuals have the time and resources to carry out their job. Higher work demands are associated with higher levels of stress.
- *Influence*   The extent to which individuals are able to contribute to decision making at work. Low levels of influence are associated with higher levels of stress.

- *Role conflict*   The extent to which individuals receive conflicting instructions from others about their work. High levels of role conflict are associated with higher levels of stress.
- *Feedback*   The extent to which individuals receive feedback about their work performance. Low levels of feedback are associated with higher levels of stress.

These, and two additional work-related factors, are discussed below:

- *Autonomy and control*   The extent to which individuals believe they can work in their own way without constant consultation. Lower levels of autonomy and control are associated with higher levels of stress
- *Social support*   The extent to which individuals feel they are supported by and rely on their colleagues at work. Lower levels of support are associated with higher levels of stress.

The main work-related factor associated with stress for all seven occupational groups in NHS trusts was work demands. Managers reported that levels of work demands were higher than the other occupational groups in the NHS trusts. The following quotes give an indication of the sources of work demand:

> *I have to cover for one of my staff who is on maternity leave and in the last month I had to produce the April budgetary control report for the two divisional accountants whilst trying to manage the office and close down the accounts for the two different timetables.*

> *Stress is caused by the anxiety of achieving demands, putting pressure on my staff, and maintaining the standard day-to-day business of the department.*

The relationship between work demands and stress symptom levels was stronger for managers; a reduction in work demands resulted in a significantly greater reduction in stress than in the other occupational groups.

For all occupational groups, a perceived lack of influence over decisions made at work was a source of stress. Managers reported significantly higher levels of influence than all other groups, and, for this group, the relationship between influence and stress levels was stronger; not being able to influence decision making resulted in significantly greater increases in stress than in other occupational groups. The quotes below give some indication of why managers found a lack of influence stressful:

During a meeting, hearing that discussion concerning the future of our service and the people in it may be sealing our future, or lack of it, without any consultation with us.

Trying to manage a change of decision by my senior which had, prior to the change, involved significant impact of management time and trade union discussion. This had to be reversed and corporate management reputation was damaged.

There were two other important work-related sources of stress for managers: role conflict and lack of feedback. One manager commented that a major source of stress was:

The different expectations that other people have of my role.

Another observed:

I have no job description so I am always uncertain about what my exact role is and the parameters within which I operate.

Another commented that for her a source of stress was:

Conflicting instructions received from a manager with no clear instructions.

A work-related source of stress identified for all occupational groups was low levels of autonomy and control. The relationship between autonomy and control and stress levels was strongest among managers; those who reported low levels of autonomy and control experienced significantly greater increases in stress levels than staff in the other occupational groups. One manager commented that, for her, a solution to stress would be for the organisation to:

show trust in my and other managers' judgements. Allow me to manage my department without punitive and "knee-jerk" constraints.

where I don't have the time to devote my attention without "urgent" mundane matters getting in the way.

Low levels of social support was another source of stress for all occupational groups. The relationship between social support and stress levels was, again, strongest for managers, such that low levels of social support resulted in significantly greater increases in stress than in other occupational groups. Managers commented on aspects of their relationships with colleagues which caused stress:

I was accused by a colleague of not keeping her informed about areas of my work which have direct consequences for her. Whilst technically this was correct insofar as I had communicated directly to her only briefly (and not face to face), it was completely untrue insofar as her nominated representative had been party to all of relevance . . . He hadn't communicated to her, although my understanding was that his sole reason for existence was liaison between us.

Trying to resolve conflicts caused by a difficult, unpredictable members of staff. Relationship problems are always the most difficult problems to work with . . . Decreased resources and increased workload mean there is no flexibility left to change the structure, therefore confrontations take place.

FEMALE MANAGERS

In the late 1980s, as the proportion of women in the labour force increased, the focus of research on managers shifted to an interest in differences in the prevalence of stress among female and male managers, and whether the factors associated with stress differed (Davidson and Cooper, 1993). Conflicting evidence exists as to whether stress among women managers is higher than among men (e.g. Van Der Pompe and De Hens, 1993). However, there is considerable agreement that female managers are exposed to a wider range of potential stressors.

McDonald and Korabik (1991) compared reports that women and men in low- and high-stress groups gave of stressors and ways of coping with stress. They found that women were more likely to identify prejudice and discrimination, and work/family interface as sources of stress. Davidson and Cooper (1993) reported the same sources of stress in their study of female managers, but identified additional stressors such as being at a lower management level than men, and lack of role models of the same sex. Korabik and Van Kampen (1995) studied the influence of sex and gender-role orientation on social support and coping with occupational stress among a sample of female and male managers. They found that women managers reported being subject to significantly more job stressors than men in comparable positions, experiencing more problems than their male counterparts due to prejudice and discrimination, negative stereotyping and social isolation.

There is also evidence that female managers' experience of their role is substantially different from their male counterparts. Pretty *et al.* (1992) reported that female managers were more sensitive to the interactions of their staff in getting the job done, while male managers were more sensitive to the demands of their senior colleagues. In addition, women were more vulnerable with respect to relationship experiences, peer cohesion, and more often gained personal accomplishment from opportunities to innovate and variety in their jobs.

Despite extensive literature searches no research studies on female health care managers were identified. The Borrill et al. (1998) study, however, found no overall gender differences in the prevalence of stress for male and female health care managers, but, in common with other studies, found that there were differences in the reported work-related sources of stress. For both female and male managers, work demands, lack of influence over decision making and role conflict were the main factors associated with stress. Additional factors for male managers were lack of support from their own managers and professional compromise (i.e. the extent to which they felt they were compromising professional standards to meet cost objectives).

Among female managers, low levels of social support, lack of feedback on performance and lack of role clarity (i.e. the extent to which individuals fully understand the duties and responsibilities expected of them) were additional work-related sources of stress. The relationship between role clarity and stress was strongest for female managers; lack of role clarity resulted in a significantly greater increase in stress for female managers than for male managers.

THE PREVALENCE OF STRESS AMONG DIFFERENT GRADES OF MANAGERS

Staff working at different levels within an organisation have differing role requirements, functions and spans of control. There is evidence that these different requirements are associated with different stressors, resulting in varying levels of stress. Stansfield and Marmot (1992) found the prevalence of stress was higher among civil servants in lower employment grades. A comparison of female managers and clerical workers reported by Long (1998) showed that the latter were more distressed and less satisfied than the managers, had fewer coping resources, appraised stress events as less controllable, and experienced more work demands and less support.

Borrill et al. (1998) examined whether the prevalence of stress and work-related factors associated with stress varied across the different management grades in NHS trusts. Managers were divided into four groups: junior/first line managers (pay scales A&C grade 6 or SMP 30–15), middle managers (A&C grade 7 or SMP 14–8), senior administrators (those on A&C grade 8 and above who reported substantial responsibility

for managing staff); and senior managers (SMP 1–7). Significant variations in the prevalence of stress across these four groups were found, as
shown in Table 8.3.

The prevalence of stress was significantly higher among junior
managers.

There are no significant differences in the work-related factors associated
with stress across grade. However, middle and junior/first line managers
reported significantly higher work demands than senior managers ($p =<$
0.05). Middle and senior managers reported higher levels of influence over
decision making than junior managers, and senior managers reported significantly higher levels of social support. Comments made by junior and
middle managers illustrate the sources of stress they experienced:

> *As myself and my colleagues are managers at a level or two below the
> trust board we tend to see much that is decided at this level which
> creates unnecessary work and expense—this as much as anything
> causes frustration in our jobs.*

> *A boss who has not wished/been able to support the work I am supposed
> to do when it is clear to him that others are deliberately undermining it.*

Table 8.3:   The prevalence of stress among different grades of manager

Grade	Number	% Stress*
Junior managers	448	36.2
Senior administrators	249	29.3
Senior managers	134	29.1
Middle managers	163	27.0

* Stress was measured using the GHQ-12 (Goldberg, 1972)

COMPARISONS BETWEEN NON-CLINICAL AND CLINICAL MANAGERS

A major recent change in health care has been the increasing involvement
of senior professional staff in management. It is a requirement that all
NHS trusts have a representative of the medical and nursing profession
as an Executive member of the Trust Board, and in the majority of trusts
professional staff take major responsibility for managing directorates and
departments in collaboration with managers. Given the range of responsibilities is different for clinical managers and managers, comparisons
were made between these two groups, examining whether the prevalence
of stress and work-related sources of stress are different.

No significant differences in the prevalence of stress for non-clinical managers and clinical managers were found, and the sources of stress were similar for these two groups. However, differences were observed between clinical and non-clinical managers in the strength of the relationship between some of the work-related factors and stress. For the non-clinical managers:

- high levels of work demands resulted in a significantly higher level of stress;
- low levels of support from their own manager resulted in a significantly greater increase in stress;
- when they perceived low levels of social support, this resulted in a significantly higher levels of stress;
- high levels of role conflict resulted in significantly higher levels of stress.

Taking these findings together suggests that non-clinical managers experienced a greater vulnerability to stressors than clinical managers. This may be because, for the latter group, clinical necessity and professional identity provided a clarity and support in their managerial role which is not available to non-clinical managers.

INTERVENTIONS TO REDUCE STRESS

This chapter has focused on the work and organisational sources of stress for health care managers. The literature reviewed highlights the wide range of potential stressors inherent in the manager's role, which are likely to be more prevalent in complex public sector organisations. There is convincing evidence that the prevalence of stress is substantially higher among health care managers than among their counterparts in other organisations, and that it is higher than among staff in other occupational groups in health care. The lack of research literature on health care managers, however, suggests that the specific problem of stress within this group of staff has gone largely unrecognised.

The research findings discussed in this chapter suggest that interventions to address the issue of stress among health care managers need to focus on both the organisational context and work role factors. That is, to take account of the factors in public sector organisations which promote the discordance, disjunction and conflict that "prevent managers from managing" Kouzes and Mico (1979, p. 464), and the specific work-related factors inherent in the complex managerial role. A range of intervention strategies are required which can increase managers' control and support and decrease conflicts and demands. Offerman and Armitage (1993) argue that stress interventions should simultaneously be targeted at three levels: individual (person-oriented interventions); work role and organisation (organisationally oriented interventions); and organisation environment (systematically oriented interventions).

Person-oriented interventions

These interventions focus on enabling managers to develop the ability to recognise the symptoms of their own stress, and to develop individual strategies for coping with stress. Maynard (1996) investigated differences in the use of counselling services across occupational groups in the NHS. She concluded that managers did not seek help when they experienced stress, primarily because they failed to recognise that they were stressed. In addition, she identified a variety of attitudinal and cultural factors which prevented managers from seeking help, even if they acknowledged that this might be beneficial. Thus, before individually-focused stress interventions are introduced for health care managers, steps need to be taken to help them to recognise the symptoms of stress and to seek help.

Organisationally oriented interventions

These fall into three main categories: job-design and redesign; support mechanisms; and organisational policy changes. Existing evidence suggests that, by improving job design, by increasing control and support, and by decreasing demands, psychological and physiological health can improve and be cost-effective (Ilgen, 1990).

Borrill et al. (1998) identified a number of work role factors specifically related to managerial stress which have implications for work design and redesign: managers reported significantly higher work demands than other groups of staff in the NHS; lower work demands among managers resulted in a greater improvement in stress than for other groups of NHS staff; lack of influence over decision making and lack of autonomy and control resulted in significantly greater increases in stress than for other groups of staff. Thus, managers who are working under considerable pressure, experience higher levels of stress than other occupational groups when they are unable to perform tasks which are critical to the successful execution of this role: making decisions and acting autonomously. Interventions to address these issues could include measures to clarify objectives and responsibilities, and reviews of decision-making and communication processes in the organisation.

Borrill et al. (1998) also found evidence that measures to improve support mechanisms for managers could also potentially reduce stress. Lack of social support, and lack of support from their own manager, resulted in significantly higher levels of stress among managers than among other occupational groups. A management development intervention carried out by Haynes *et al.* (reported in Borrill *et al.*, 1998), included managers attending management skills workshops. Managers reported benefits from the opportunity to discuss and reflect on current work practices with colleagues in similar jobs, and to learn from each others' experiences.

Work demands, lack of influence, role conflict and lack of feedback were identified as sources of stress for all NHS occupational groups; however, among managers, there was a stronger relationship between these factors and stress. Intuitively, managers who are overloaded with work, who feel that they have little or no influence over decisions which affect them, who are unsure of their key responsibilities, and who receive little or no feedback (either positive or negative) will be less likely to be able to provide managerial support to staff. Therefore, an organisation considering investing in interventions to reduce stress would benefit from targeting managers in the first instance.

In addition, the focus on managers must also take account of the differing needs and experiences of male and female managers reported above. For example, Borrill *et al.* (1998) found that male managers report lack of leader support and professional compromise as unique stressors, whereas female managers report that lack of social support, lack of feedback and lack of role clarity are associated with stress.

Murphy (1995, and see Chapter 11) provides comprehensive, practical guidelines for planning and implementing stress management interventions at these levels, including advice on evaluation and process.

Systematically oriented interventions

These are the intervention approaches which relate to the organisational environment. Earlier in the chapter, discussion focused on public/private sector management role differences, and concluded that public sector managers may be exposed to a wider range of organisational and work-related sources of stress than their private sector counterparts. Intervention by national governments in the area of work stress among health care managers has never been more critical, particularly given their key role in setting national policies and procedures for health care systems. Traditionally, in both the government and academic sectors, it has been the well-being of professionals, mainly nurses and doctors, who receive the most public scrutiny.

The impact that government policy can have on health services and the staff working within them was recognised by the managers in the Borrill *et al.* (1998) study:

The fast changing of the NHS causes extreme demands on finance departments. The trust is lacking in planning for these changes, new training/development needs. People are being pushed into sink or swim, and faced with the front line positions new to them without appropriate support and training.

The reforms of the NHS need to be made with firm timetables and guidance. Allow good organisations to progress services. Minimise central interference with ministers setting strategic direction and standards only.

The economic success and efficient functioning of health services are as dependent on their managers as on their clinical professionals' expertise and vigilance. Moreover, since the introduction of clinical governance in addition to financial governance, the quality of care provided is also their ultimate responsibility. For this reason, continued and increasing government awareness of the possible stressors faced by managers in health care is essential. Future initiatives should be designed to target and support this group with the aim of improving their well-being.

REFERENCES

Borrill, C.S., Wall, T.D., West, M.A., Hardy, G.E., Carter, A.J., Haynes, C.E., Shapiro, D.A., Stride, C. and Wood, D. (1998). *Stress among NHS Staff: Final Report.* Institute of Work Psychology, Sheffield University.

Burke, R.J. (1988). Sources of managerial and professional stress in large organisations. In C.L. Cooper and R. Payne (Eds) *Causes, Coping and Consequences of Stress at Work.* New York: Wiley.

Caplan, R. (1994) Stress, anxiety, and depression in hospital consultants, general practitioners, and senior health service managers. *British Medical Journal,* **309**, 1261–1263.

Cooper, C.L. and Marshall, J. (1978). *Understanding Executive Stress.* London: Macmillan.

Cooper, C.L. and Melhuish, A. (1984) Executive stress and health: differences between men and women. *Journal of Occupational Medicine,* **26**, 2, 99–104.

Cooper, C.L., Sloan, S.J. and Williams, S. (1988). *Occupational Stress Indicator Management Guide.* Windsor: NFER-Nelson.

Davidson, M.J. and Cooper, C.L. (1993). *Shattering the Glass Ceiling. The Woman Manager.* London: Paul Chapman.

Gill, J. and Foulder, I. (1978). Managing a merger: the acquisition and its aftermath. *Personnel Management,* **10**, 14–17.

Goldberg, D.P., (1972). *The Detection of Minor Psychiatric Illness by Questionnaire.* Oxford: Oxford University Press.

Hirschorn, L. (1983). *Cutting Back.* San Francisco: Jossey-Bass.

Hunt, J.W. (1986). Alienation among managers: the new epidemic or the social scientists' invention? *Personnel Review,* **15**, 21–6.

Ilgen D. (1990). Health issues at work: industrial-organisational psychology opportunities. *American Psychologist*, **45**, 273–283.

Jick, T.D. (1983). The stressful effects of budget cuts in organisations. In L.A. Rosen (Ed.) *Topics in Managerial Accounting*. New York: McGraw-Hill.

Korabik, K. and Van Kampen, J. (1995) Gender, social support, and coping with work stressers among managers. *Journal of Social Behaviour and Personality*, **10**(6), 135–148.

Kouzes, J.M. and Mico, P.R. (1979) Domain theory, an introduction to organisational behaviour in human service organisations. *Journal of Applied Behavioural Science*, **15**(4), 449–469.

Litwinenko, A. and Cooper, C.L. (1995). The impact of trust status on health care workers. *Journal of Managerial Psychology*, **10**, 3.

Long, B.C. (1998) Coping with workplace stress: a multiple-group comparison of female managers and clerical workers. *Journal of Counselling Psychology*, **45**(1), 65–78.

Maynard, L. (1996). Mental health support for senior NHS managers. *Occupational Health*, **48**(7), 243–246.

McDonald, L.M. and Korabik, K. (1991). Sources of stress and ways of coping among male and female managers. *Journal of Social Behaviour and Personality*, **6**(7), 185–198.

Mullarkey, S., Wall, T.D., Clegg, C.W. and Warr, P.B. (1998). *Measures of Strain, Job Satisfaction and Job-related Well-being: A Manual of Normative Data*. Institute of Work Psychology, University of Sheffield (in preparation).

Murphy, L.R. (1995). Occupational stress management: current status and future directions. In C.L. Cooper and D.M. Rousseau (Eds) *Trends in Organizational Behavior*, Vol. 2. Chichester: Wiley.

Offerman, L.R. and Armitage, M.A. (1993). Stress and the woman manager: sources, health outcomes and interventions. In E.A. Fagenson (Ed.) *Women in Management: Trends, Issues and Challenges in Managerial Diversity*. Newbury Park, CA: Sage.

Pretty, G.M.H., McCarthy, M.E. and Catano, U.M. (1992). Psychological environments and burnout: gender consideration within the corporation. *Journal of Organisational Behaviour*, **13**, 701–711.

Salaman, G.S. (1995). *Managing*. Buckingham: Open University Press.

Stansfield, S.A. and Marmot, M.G. (1992). Social class and minor psychiatric disorder in British Civil Servants: a validated screening survey using the General Health Questionnaire. *Psychological Medicine*, **22**, 739–749.

Turnage, J.J. and Spielberger, C.D. (1991). Job stress in managers, professionals, and clinical workers. *Work and Stress*, **5**(3), 165–176.

Van Der Pompe, G. and De Hens, P. (1993). Work stress, social support, and strains among male and female managers. *Anxiety, Stress and Coping*, **6**, 215–229.

Wall, T.D., Bolden, R.I., Borrill, C.S., Carter, A.J., Golya, D.A., Hardy, G.E., Haynes, C.E., Rick, J.E., Shapiro, D.A. and West, M.A. (1997). Minor psychiatric disorder in NHS trust staff: occupational and gender differences. *British Journal of Psychiatry*, **171**, 519–523.

West, M.A., Lawthom, R., Patterson, M. and Staniforth, D. (1995). *Still Far to Go: The Management of UK Manufacturing*, Institute of Work Psychology, Sheffield University.

Wolpin, I. and Burke, R.J. (1986). Occupational locking-in: some correlates and consequences, *International Review of Applied Psychology*, **35**, 327–345.

9

STRESS IN AMBULANCE PERSONNEL

Kathryn M. Young and Cary L. Cooper

> *The Ambulance Service is thus a stressful occupation but nevertheless a rewarding one.*
> JAMES (1988)

INTRODUCTION

Ambulance personnel are among the highest risk group of health care staff for stress and burnout (Hammer *et al.*, 1986; James, 1988; Grigsby and McKnew, 1988; Mitchell, 1984). The Association of Chief Ambulance Officers (Ambulance 2000, 1990) concluded that the high levels of early ill-health retirements and death observed in the Service were attributable to stress. Miletich (1990) suggested from the literature that responding to incidents which were difficult, dangerous, potentially life threatening and under both public scrutiny and potential threat from hostility and verbal abuse was intrinsically stressful to ambulance personnel. Grigsby and McKnew (1988) went further, proposing that it is the responsibility for human health and life which influences the high levels of stress which impact on the health and well-being of paramedic staff. Sutherland and Cooper (1990) point to the huge costs to the individual, industry and society of mismanaged stress. But are the high levels of stress observed in ambulance personnel a result of intrinsic and inherent sources of stress in ambulance work or stress outcomes mismanaged by employers?

Stress in Health Professionals. Edited by Jenny Firth-Cozens and Roy L. Payne
© 1999 John Wiley & Sons Ltd

In order to gain a better understanding of how the sources of pressure, the stressors identified in ambulance work, might actually relate to the negative psychological consequences inferred, the stress process itself needs to be considered.

SOURCES OF STRESS IN AMBULANCE WORK

The approach commonly taken to investigate the apparent stressful nature of ambulance work has been the stimulus approach which has led to the identification of sources of pressure in ambulance work which may influence ill-health outcomes in personnel. Mason (1982) investigated stress in paramedics using a series of self-report measures. Three specific stressors in ambulance work were identified; infant death, mass casualties and childbirth with complications. Hammer *et al.* (1986) used the Medical Personnel Stress Survey—Revised and found higher levels of stress in paramedic staff than in other hospital employees. The sources of observed stress were categorised in four ways: organisational, job dissatisfaction, attitude regarding patients and somatic distress. Mitchell (1984) investigated two categories of work-related stressors in a sample of paramedics, administrative factors and clinical factors, and found administrative factors to be the more important.

While these studies have produced evidence of pressure, James (1988) went further, examining the relationships between a range of measurable constructs in 250 British ambulance personnel. Stressor items, their perceived importance and a series of mediating variables (e.g. personality characteristics, such as locus of control and demographic information) was assessed A four-factor model of ambulance staff's perception of sources of stress emerged: organisation and management aspects; new, unfamiliar and difficult duties/uncertainty; work overload; and interpersonal relations. Multiple regression analysis revealed the relationships between the factors extracted and the moderator variables measured. Seven per cent of the variance in perceptions of stressors by management and organisation factors were accounted for by scores on the "powerful others" subcale of the locus of control measure. People who believe that powerful others control their fate were more likely to see stress from this source. The other three factors were explained slightly more successfully by length of service, "chance" and "powerful others". Increased perceptions of stress were related to having a shorter length of service and attributing control over what goes on in the workplace to chance and powerful others, which may be described as a more "external" locus of control. James and Wright (1991) re-examined the sources of stress in ambulance work and concluded that the major sources were "extrinsic to the job", citing the way personnel were treated by other people as an example. However, limitations in their questionnaire design were later recognised and they suggested an underestimation of the role of "intrinsic" sources of stress, such as dealing with patients. Glendon and Glendon (1992) also aimed to identify sources of stress for ambulance personnel using a questionnaire comprising 110 items derived from in-depth interview responses. Factor analysis of their data from 184 respondents yielded six factors, of which the top four were considered congruent with the findings of James (1988). The two additional factors were described as "domestic" and "driving" stressors.

An alternative approach, namely an exploratory qualitative study was undertaken by Sparrius (1992) to identify occupational stressors occurring in ambulance and rescue service workers. Organisation-based stressors were found to be the most important, specifically with regard to the organisational design, style of management, and the disciplinary system. This emphasis on organisation-based stressors may result from the particular sample of staff obtained, as almost half of the respondents, 9 out of 20 staff, were trainees with less than six months' service. However, a small-scale study conducted in the UK by Hamill (1991) also found support for organisational factors being the greatest source of pressure.

A more comprehensive study of the stressor–stress relationship was undertaken by Thompson and Suzuki (1991) in a sample of 40 qualified ambulance personnel in the London Ambulance Service. A six-part questionnaire was used which comprised a scale to measure the frequency and perceived stress of 10 types of emergency call; the Impact of Events Scale (Horowitz et al., 1979), the 28-item version of the GHQ (Goldberg and Hillier, 1979), a modified Ways of Coping Questionnaire (Lazarus and Folkman, 1984), sections for behavioural and emotional indicators of stress, and other qualitative data. A list of 10 types of emergency call were identified using structured interviews in which participants assessed the perceived frequency and stressfulness of each type of call. Calls involving children, disaster incidents, and major fires, all of which occurred the least frequently, were associated with higher levels of perceived pressure. A major limitation of this study was the emphasis on emergency calls as the only source of pressure for ambulance personnel.

Young and Cooper (1995) carried out a diagnostic study of organisational stress in ambulance personnel and compared their findings with a group of firefighters. The authors based their study on an interactive model of stress and used the Occupational Stress Indicator (OSI) devised by Cooper et al. (1988) to measure seven different aspects of the stressor–stress relationship in a sample of 427 emergency workers. The sources of stress at work were measured on the sources of job pressure scale of the

OSI. Cooper *et al.*'s (1988) model proposes that sources of stress in the workplace can effectively be classified under six main headings: "factors intrinsic to the job itself, role stress specifically from the managerial role, interpersonal relationships, career and achievement, the organisational structure and climate, and the home and work interface". Significantly more job pressure was perceived by both ambulance personnel and fire-fighters than other comparable occupational groups, but the amount and sources of pressure differed across services. Ambulance personnel reported significantly more pressure from two factors: "career and achievement" and the "organisational structure and climate", but significantly less pressure from "factors intrinsic to ambulance work"; while firefighters perceived only their "relationships with others" to be a significantly greater source of pressure. Comparing the services showed that pressure from the "organisational structure and climate" was greater for ambulance personnel, (mean 43.73, sd 9.21; mean 40.74, sd 8.49; $t = 2.86$, $p<0.001$) while "relationships with other people" produced more pressure for firefighters. (mean 31.21, sd 7.22; mean 33.57, sd 7.51; $t = 2.83$, $p<0.001$).

Young (1995) conducted a longitudinal study of stress in ambulance personnel over an 18-month period following the industrial dispute which took place in the UK ambulance service in 1989–90. Data were collected using the OSI at the time of the dispute, during the restructuring of the service, and during the implementation of a new operational structure. A changing pattern of sources of pressure and the underlying consistent sources were revealed.

The structure and climate of the ambulance service, and lack of opportunities for achievement and advancement at work, were found to present continual, high-level sources of pressure. Perceived pressures from the "managerial role", "relationships with others at work" and the "home and work relationship" were found to fluctuate over time. However, ambulance work itself as a source of pressure, which had not been high during the dispute, produced much less pressure in the phases that followed.

What all these studies demonstrate quite clearly is that sources other than ambulance work itself produce pressure for ambulance personnel, which would not be the case if it were inherently stressful. Nevertheless, some aspects of the job, such as incidents involving children, are shown to be more problematic than others. The high levels of perceived pressure reported may be attributed to organisational sources of pressure and confirms what Brown and Campbell (1991) observe in the emergency services in general: that "management and organisational aspects of the emergency services are more frequently sources of stress than operational duties".

INDIVIDUAL CHARACTERISTICS OF AMBULANCE PERSONNEL

The interactional approach to stress proposes that situations of themselves are not necessarily stressful: the level of stress depends upon the interaction between the individual and the situation. Two of the most widely researched individual characteristics have been the Type A behaviour pattern and locus of control.

The Type A behaviour pattern

The Type A behaviour pattern, first identified by Dunbar (1943), is characterised by compulsive striving, self-discipline, an urge to get to the top and have mastery over others. Two studies report the influence of the Type A behaviour pattern in ambulance personnel and suggest that the levels of this style of behaviour observed would not generally influence stress outcomes.Young and Cooper (1995) used the Type A scale of the OSI to measure the extent of this behaviour pattern, and also compared the findings with firefighters. The amount of Type A behaviour, overall, was not significantly high in either service. Young and Cooper (1998), in their longitudinal study of ambulance personnel, found that the amount of Type A behaviour remained at a consistent and acceptable level over time, showing that a stable trait was being measured by the OSI.

Locus of control

The concept of locus of control (Rotter, 1966) refers to the extent to which an individual perceives that he or she has control over a given situation, generally being defined as "power" or "mastery" over the environment and has close links with the concept of competence. In addition to the study by James (1988) described above, Young and Cooper (1995) measured locus of control using the relevant scale of the OSI, in their comparisons of ambulance personnel and firefighters. Staff in both services revealed significantly more "externality" than the norm and externality was correlated with job satisfaction, symptoms of mental health and physical ill-health. The longitudinal study of ambulance personnel conducted by Young and Cooper (1999) included measures of locus of control over time. Unlike the more constant pattern of Type A behaviour, locus of control was found to change significantly over time, specifically towards increased "externality". This may make individuals more predisposed to the effects of stress.

The work of Paulhus and Christie (1981) on domains, provides a particularly cogent explanation of why a disproportionate amount of "externals" are found in these two emergency services. The type of work that both ambulance personnel and firefighters undertake may be broadly described as reversing negative or hazardous environments. The demand to act, once a 999 call is received, is immediate. Staff receive skills training and there are often set procedures and protocols to be followed. Importantly, feedback on both successful and non-successful action is often rapid. Satisfaction would occur when there was more positive feedback than negative, and even in the case of failure, credit would be given for trying. This exercise of control over aspects of the environment may be the powerful motivating force which sustains staff in emergency work, and may be the source of their reported satisfaction. It also suggests that emergency staff may generally be able to exercise control in one domain only, that of their own job tasks, where we know they perceive far less pressure. The influence of "externality" then becomes apparent in other domains at work where they perceive less ability to exert influence.

THE COPING TECHNIQUES USED BY AMBULANCE PERSONNEL

Coping can be seen as a preventive strategy rather than just a reaction; an effective means of reducing work stress if it is anticipated. This preventive aspect of coping can be seen among the strategies that Palmer (1983) identifies in paramedics dealing with death and dying. A participant observation approach was used during approximately 500 hours spent with emergency medical technicians. Six principal coping aids were identified: (1) the educational desensitisation process, which serves to reduce fear and helplessness; (2) use of humour; (3) language alternation, which involves using technical language or argot; (4) scientific fragmentation and escape into work such as referring to patients by their symptoms, for example, the miscarriage; and (5) rationalisation, the recognition that death may be a relief from suffering.

Thompson and Suzuki (1991) used a modified version of the Ways of Coping Questionnaire (Lazarus and Folkman, 1984) to assess how ambulance personnel were attempting to cope with perceived pressure at work. The most routinely used coping technique was self-control, along with escape/avoidance, distancing and planful problem solving. This study shows that ambulance personnel tend to use alternative coping techniques to what the stress literature maintains is a most effective means for reducing the effects of stress, namely, utilising social support.

Supportive social relationships have been conceptualised as operating in three ways to alleviate the effects of stress: directly enhancing health, reducing interpersonal tensions, and acting as a buffering or interactional effect. The OSI "sources of coping scale" used by Young and Cooper (1995) to investigate the coping behaviour of ambulance personnel, included social support among its six subscales and allowed the use of this technique to be compared with others. As expected, particular coping techniques were used significantly more or less frequently to manage the pressures at work. In particular, greater reliance was placed on the "home and work relationship", which was also found to be the case for firefighters. In addition, ambulance personnel were found to use "logic" more frequently and "social support" much less often.

Young and Cooper (1999) examined how the amount and type of coping behaviours changed over time in a cohort of ambulance personnel and found major fluctuations. Increasing reliance on the "home and work relationship" was found, that is, focusing outside the workplace for support. In contrast, increasingly less use was made of social support *within* work, along with less "involvement" in the issues causing pressure at work. LaRocco and Jones (1978) identified "the team" as a prime source of social support and a buffer against the negative effects of job stress, but the studies cited above show that ambulance personnel generally fail to seek social support at work.

Beaton *et al.* (1997), in samples of paramedics and firefighters, tested both the buffering hypothesis—that social support mediates against the effects of job-related stressors—and the costs of non-support hypothesis—that is, that conflicting social relationships negatively influence stress outcomes. Support was found for both hypotheses: social support and relational conflict with co-workers directly influenced respondents' appraisal of sources of stress at work. The subsequent effects on self-reported job satisfaction, and stress symptom health outcome measures were also demonstrated.

These studies show that ambulance personnel and, to a lesser extent, firefighters adopt strategies of avoidance and self-control; fail to get involved with the issues causing pressure; focus outside the work environment; and, most importantly, fail to mobilise social support. This suggests dealing with pressure at work by disengaging rather than confronting the sources of pressure, which may have a negative impact on their experience of stress.

James (1988) points out that ambulance work gives personnel a particular view of society as it requires them to deal with people in difficulties, in states of panic, distress and shock. In the workplace they are also subject to threat from disease, potential violence from patients and from members of the public. Indeed, Mezey and Shepherd (1994) report that not only are health care workers, including ambulance staff, at particularly high risk from assault at work, but actual assaults are common. In addition, Talbot *et al.* (1992) found that dealing with violent death and injury, routine for ambulance personnel engaged full-time in accident and emergency work, can trigger awareness of an individual's own mortality, personal vulnerability and survivor guilt. All these threats constitute challenges to the schemas that are held by individuals to account for how the world works, and require responses to them.

Acute stress occurs at the point at which events experienced by a person present major challenges sufficient to cause a breakdown of coping strategies. Attempting to cope with them can give rise to the intrusive thoughts, imagery and avoidance commonly associated with post-traumatic stress disorder (PTSD). The term is commonly used to refer to the reactions of a small proportion of people, around 1.5% in the general population (Rick et al., 1998), in the aftermath of an extreme incident. These reactions are characterised by intrusion, persistently re-experiencing the event, avoidance of reminders of the event, and hyper-arousal or increased startle response (DSM IV, APA, 1994). The development of both chronic stress and PTSD would therefore result from failure to integrate the experience.

Avoidance is a strategy for dealing with anxiety and fear and is commonly used by ambulance personnel. Janoff-Bulman and Timko (1987) identify both avoidance of reminders of an event and denial as potentially adaptive coping strategies serving to control the initial impact of events and allow a more gradual process of integration. However, Folkman and Lazarus (1986) suggest that while such "emotion-focused" coping may be effective in the short term, suppressing emotion in the long term may impair adaptation, or integration, by interfering with the cognitive function. This "cognitive function" would necessarily be the process required to rebuild the shattered "assumptive world". It would seem, then, that such a strategy for perceiving incidents may have short-term benefits but long-term negative consequences for ambulance personnel.

Kilpatrick et al. (1982) and Keane et al. (1985) offer an explanation based on avoidance strategies to account for the failure of ambulance personnel to use social support as a coping strategy. They suggest that the need to avoid talking about, and thereby re-experiencing, stressful events may be greater than the desire to integrate the trauma experience. They propose a link between failure to exploit social support as a coping strategy and the development and maintenance of PTSD.

THE EFFECTS OF STRESS ON AMBULANCE PERSONNEL

Health outcomes of stress

Until the early 1980s, there was little or no recognition that emergency workers, including ambulance personnel, could experience mental and

physical ill-health outcomes as a result of their work. The first indications
of psychological distress came from Taylor and Frazer (1982) who studied
rescue workers following a disaster. Since then, the effects of stress in
terms of health outcomes have been well recognised in emergency service
personnel (Jones, 1985; Duckworth, 1986; Shepherd and Hodgkinson,
1990) prompting the view of disaster rescue workers as secondary victims. McFarlane (1989) found that factors predisposing ill-health outcomes were the same for both disaster survivors and helpers, the
secondary victims. Mitchell (1984) also found civilians and emergency
workers equally susceptible to physical and psychological responses to
trauma.

Ravenscroft (1993) conducted a survey of ill-health outcomes in personnel in the London Ambulance Service using an unidentified measure of
traumatic stress symptoms related to PTSD and the General Health Questionnaire (GHQ). A prevalence of 15% of personnel reporting above
threshold symptoms for PTSD was found compared with the 1–1.5%
found generally, while 53% were found to be over the threshold for
emotional distress or "caseness" as measured by the GHQ. Thompson
and Suzuki (1991) also examined levels of perceived stress in ambulance
personnel using both traumatic stress and general ill-health measures.
The Impact of Events Scale (IES; Horowitz et al, 1979) was used to measure the amount of intrusive imagery associated with a recent event and
the degree of subsequent avoidance behaviour. "Intrusion" was found to
be a particular problem although less severe than the clinical population.
General stress was measured using the GHQ (28-item version). Results
confirmed the findings of Ravenscroft (1993) with 60% of the sample
achieving scores higher than the usual cut-off of 5 and above, indicating
probable psychological distress or "caseness". Taking a higher cut-off
point of 12, showed 20% of the sample manifesting high levels of symp-
tomatic distress.

The types of incident Ravenscroft found to influence PTSD outcomes
were smaller scale, routine incidents such as cot death and injured or
dead children rather than major events such as the Clapham Rail Crash
and the King's Cross Fire. This is partially in line with Thompson and
Suzuki (1991) who found that emergency calls involving children were
perceived as being the most stressful. These potentially distressing and
disturbing incidents are a continuous feature of ambulance work, unlike
the discrete major incident.

Two studies on health outcomes of stress using the interactional approach were carried out by Young and Cooper (1995, 1999). These studies
established the severity of the problem for ambulance personnel and also
determined the influences on health outcomes at one point in time and an
observed negative change in the mental health over time. In the first,

Young and Cooper (1995) measured health outcomes for ambulance personnel using the mental and physical health scales of the OSI. The mental health scale consists of items related to psycho-neurotic symptoms and the physical health scale to psycho-somatic symptoms. Evidence of poor mental and physical health was influenced by different and wide-ranging variables. The mental ill-health of ambulance personnel was influenced by perceived pressure from "relations with other people", the "style of behaviour" generally exhibited and their failure to utilise coping techniques. The high level of physical ill-health in ambulance personnel was influenced by: perceived pressure from their "relations with other people"; their inability to exert "individual influence" and "style of behaviour".

Change in mental and physical health over time was investigated by Young and Cooper (1999). The amount of physical ill-health reported by ambulance personnel showed no appreciable change over time, but a perceived inability to exert individual influence was predictive of an increase in the symptoms of mental ill-health.

These studies all confirm severe ill-health outcomes of stress in ambulance personnel and levels of physical ill-health, comparable with that of firefighters, which are not related to factors associated with ambulance work itself.

EFFECTS OF STRESS FOR THE AMBULANCE SERVICE

The chief organisational effect of stress in ambulance personnel is that of sickness absence. Toombs et al. (1979) investigated occupational stress factors in the London Ambulance Service and found a high rate of sickness absence, a proportion of which was judged to be stress-related. Stilwell and Stilwell (1984) compared the sickness absence records of ambulance and fire staff and found slightly higher rates of absence for ambulance staff than for fire staff, and higher rates among female ambulance staff. The chief reason for the high level of sickness absence reported by ambulance staff recorded on medical certificates was musculo-skeletal injury. Glendon and Glendon (1992) used a self-report questionnaire to investigated sickness absence in ambulance personnel and reported findings comparable with those of Stilwell and Stilwell (1984). Young (1995) also investigated self-reported sickness absence as an organisational outcome of stress and found much higher levels than those reported by the previous authors. Almost 50% of ambulance personnel reported sickness absence of over 10 days in the previous year, which was comparable to that of firefighters. A further addition in this study was a measure of attribution for absence, with 37% of ambulance personnel attributed their absence to a job-related cause, more than double that for fire-fighters. Attempts were made to determine the influences on the high level of sickness absence observed, but the variables measured in this study, sources of pressure, individual characteristics and coping techniques, largely failed to account for the absences. It may be that pressure from the number of stressful events encountered during the course of their duties influence sickness absence, as we know from this study that around 75% of ambulance personnel had recently encountered events of a stressful nature. Sickness absence and ill-health retirement are very costly for ambulance services and, wherever possible, absence which can be attributed to a stress-related cause should be minimised with appropriate stress management strategies.

This review has provided evidence of major stress outcomes for ambulance personnel, low job satisfaction, poor mental and physical health and high levels of sickness absence, and demonstrated that influences other than ambulance work itself may be responsible. The challenge is to develop strategies to manage psycho-social stress in the service.

REFERENCES

Ambulance 2000 (1990). *Proposals for the Future Development of the Ambulance Service.* (Ringwood: Association of Chief Ambulance Officers.

Beaton, R.D., Murphy, S.A., Pike, K.C. and Corneil, W. (1997). Social support and network conflict in firefighters and paramedics. *Western Journal of Nursing Research*, **19**(3), 297–313.

Brown, J.M. and Campbell. E.A. (1991). Stress among emergency service personnel: progress and problems. *Journal of the Society for Occupational Medicine*, **41**.

Cooper, C.L., Sloan, S.J. and Williams, S. (1988). *Occupational Stress Indicator: Management Guide.* Kent: Hodder & Stoughton.

Duckworth, D.H. (1986). Psychological problems arising from disaster work. *Stress Medicine*, **2**, 315–323.

Dunbar, F. (1943). *Psychosomatic Medicine.* New York: Hoeber.

Folkman, S. and Lazarus, R.S. (1986). Stress processes and depressive symptomology. *Journal of Abnormal Psychology*, **95**(2), 107–113.

Glendon, A.I. and Glendon, S. (1992). Stress in ambulance staff In E.J. Lovesey (Ed.) *Contemporary Ergonomics 1992: "ergonomics for industry".* Proceedings of the Ergonomics Society's 1992 Annual Conference (pp. 174–180). Birmingham: Taylor & Francis.

Goldberg, D.P. and Hillier, V.F. (1979). A scaled version of the General Health Questionnaire. *Psychological Medicine*, **9**, 139–145.

Grigsby, D.W. and McKnew, M.A. (1988). Work-stress burnout among paramedics. *Psychological Reports*, **63**, 55–64.

Hamill, N. (1991). *Sources and levels of stress in ambulance personnel and ways of coping.* Unpublished report, Birmingham University: School of Psychology.

Hammer, J.S., Mathews, J.J., Lyons, J.S. and Johnson, N.J. (1986). Occupational stress within the paramedic profession: an initial report of stress levels compared to hospital employees. *Annals of Emergency Medicine*, 15, 536–539.

Horowitz, M.D., Wilner, N. and Alvarez, W. (1979). Impact of Event Scale: a measure of subjective stress. *Psychosomatic Medicine*, 41(3), 209–218.

James, A. (1988). Perceptions of stress in British ambulance personnel. *Work and Stress*, 2(4), 319–326.

James, A. and Wright, P.L. (1991). Occupational stress in the ambulance service. *Health Manpower Management*, 17, 4.

Janoff-Bulman, R. and Timko, C. (1987). Coping with traumatic life events: the role of denial in the light of people's assumptive worlds. In C. Snyder and C. Ford (Eds) *Coping with Negative Life Events: Clinical and Social Psychological Perspectives*. New York: Plenum.

Jones, D.R. (1985). Secondary disaster victims: the emotional effects of recovering and identifying human remains. *American Journal of Psychiatry*, 142, 3.

Keane, T.M., Scott, W.O., Chavoya, G.A. *et al.* (1985). Social support in vietnam veterans: a comparative analysis. *Journal of Consulting and Clinical Psycholog*, 53, 95–102.

Kilpatrick, D.G., Veronen, L.J. and Resick, P.A. (1982). The aftermath of rape: factors predicting successful coping at three months post-rape. Paper presented at the 59th Annual Meeting of the American Orthopsychiatric Association, San Francisco, CA.

LaRocco, J.M. and Jones, P. (1978) Co-worker and leader support as moderators of the stress–strain relationship. *Journal of Applied Psychology*, 63, 629–631.

Lazarus, R.S. and Folkman, S. (1984) Coping and adaptation. In W.D. Gentry (Ed.) *The Handbook of Behavioural Medicine*. (pp. 282–325) New York: Guilford.

Mason, J.H. (1982) Stress in paramedics. *Dissertation Abstracts International*, 43 (5-A).

McFarlane, A. (1989) The aetiology of post traumatic morbidity: pre-disposing, precipitating and perpetuating factors. *British Journal of Psychiatry*, 154, 221–228.

Mezey, G. and Shepherd, J. (1994) Effects on health care professionals. In *Violence in Health Care: A Practical Guide to Coping with Violence and Caring for Victims*. Oxford: Oxford University Press.

Miletich, J.J. (1990). Police, firefighter and paramedic stress: an annotated bibliography. *Bibliographies and Indexes in Psychology*, Number 6. New York: Greenwood Press.

Mitchell, J.T. (1984). The 600 run limit. *Journal of Emergency Medical Services*, 9(1), 52–54.

Paulhus, D. and Christie, R. (1981). Spheres of control. In H. Lefcourt (Ed.). *Research with the Locus of Control Construct, Vol.1. Assessment Methods*. New York: Academic Press.

Palmer, E. (1983). A note on paramedics' strategies for dealing with death and dying. *Journal of Occupational Psychology*, 56, 83–86.

Ravenscroft, T. (1993). *Report of a thesis into post-traumatic stress disorder in the London ambulance service*. Unpublished BSc Project, London University.

Rick, J., Perryman, S., Young, K., Guppy, A. and Hillage, J. (1998). *Workplace Trauma and its Management: Review of the Literature*. Health and Safety Executive, Contract Report 170/1988.

Rotter, J.B. (1966). Generalised expectancies for internal vs external control of reinforcement. *Psychological Monographs*, 80(1), 184–215.

Sparrius, S. (1992). Occupational stressors among ambulance and rescue service workers. *South African Journal of Psychology*, **22**(2), 87–91.

Shepherd, M. and Hodgkinson, P.E. (1990). The hidden victims of disaster: helper stress. *Medicine*, **6**, 29–35.

Stilwell, J.A. and Stilwell, P.J. (1984). Sickness absence in an ambulance service. *Journal of Social and Occupational Medicine*, **34**, 96–99.

Sutherland, V.J. and Cooper, C.L. (1990). *Understanding Stress: A Psychological Perspective for Health Professionals.* Psychology and Health Series, edited by D. Marcer. London: Chapman and Hall.

Talbot, A., Manton, M. and Dunn, P. (1992). Debriefing the debriefers. *Journal of Traumatic Stress*, **3**, 265–278.

Taylor, A.J.W. and Frazer, A.G. (1982). The stress of post disaster body handling and victim work. *Journal of Human Stress*, 4.

Thompson, J. and Suzuki, I. (1991). Stress in ambulance workers. *Disaster Management*, **3**(4), 193–197.

Toombs, F.S., Quinlan, T.P. and Terry, D.W. (1979) *Report of a Survey into Occupational Stress Factors.* London: Advisory Conciliation and Arbitration Service.

Young, K.M. (1995) *A diagnostic investigation of organisational stress in the ambulance service.* Unpublished PhD Thesis, UMIST.

Young, K.M. and Cooper, C.L. (1995). Occupational stress in the ambulance service: a diagnostic study. *Journal of Managerial Psychology*, **10**(3), 29–36.

Young, K.M. and Cooper, C. L. (1999). Change in stress outcomes following an industrial dispute in the ambulance service: a longitudinal study. *Health Services Management Research*, **12**, 51–62.

10

CHILD PROTECTION WORKERS

Tricia Cresswell and Jenny Firth-Cozens

> *I am overworked, I am spending more and more of my time in Court. The buck stops here and yet no one supports me. Managers feel that child protection is a small part of my job and one that can be squeezed on so I can take on more acute work.*
> COMMUNITY PAEDIATRICIAN

Many health professionals who deal with children and families will occasionally be required to deal with child protection issues whereas, for a relatively few, child protection is a major part of their work. In England and Wales, The Children Act 1989 established the legislative framework for child protection investigations. Local Authority Social Services Departments were given the lead responsibility for the protection of children thought to be at risk of significant harm and other agencies were required to co-operate. The major Government guidance issued at the time, *Working Together under the Children Act 1989* (Home Office, Department of Health, Department of Education and Science and the Welsh Office, 1991) stated that: *"Health professionals are major contributors to the interagency care of children that extends beyond the initial referral and assessment into child protection conference attendance, participation in planning and the ongoing support of the child and family"*.

Stress in Health Professionals. Edited by Jenny Firth-Cozens and Roy L. Payne
© 1999 John Wiley & Sons Ltd

THE HISTORICAL CONTEXT

Child abuse was either condoned or ignored until the nineteenth century (De Mause, 1976) when a number of parliamentary Acts gradually protected children in England and Wales from the extremes of wilful ill-treatment, neglect, abandonment and workplace cruelty and deprivation. By the end of the century the National Society for the Prevention of Cruelty to Children was established and Freud's controversial views, that sexual abuse was a prime cause of later psychopathology, were beginning to be discussed. Freud subsequently recast his theory to emphasise unconscious fantasy and Oedipal conflict rather than any actual sexual abuse and this theoretical U-turn has been mirrored by public opinion and policy throughout the second half of the twentieth century: what Mollon has described as a swing from seeing sexual abuse everywhere to refusing to see it at all (Mollon, 1988). Reder suggests that physical abuse of children was "rediscovered" in the 1940s and sexual abuse in the 1980s (Reder *et al.*, 1993). At the same time psychoanalytical explanations of child abuse (e.g. Kempe and Helfer, 1972) led to the development of treatment models involving the encouragement of a long-term nurturing therapeutic relationship with parents, causing confusion as to who was the client, with a focus on the welfare of parents to the possible exclusion of that of the child (Reder *et al.*, 1993).

In the 1970s and 1980s there were a series of child abuse tragedies in Britain which evoked powerful public and media response. Public inquiries into the deaths of Maria Colwell, Jasmine Beckford and Kimberley Carlile stressed the need for the protection of children when necessary by removal from their families. The Children Act 1989 was framed against this background. However, the events in Cleveland, where 82 children were the subject of place of safety orders (mostly in relation to alleged sexual abuse) in May–June 1987, led to the inquiry by Lord Justice Butler-Sloss (Cmd 412, 1988). Blame shifted once again to professionals, now accused by the media of being too ready to separate children from their families on suspicion of sexual abuse (Donaldson and O'Brien, 1995).

The Children Act reflects this potential dichotomy stating not only that the welfare of the child is paramount but also that children should (wherever possible) be brought up in their own families. As Hallet and Birchall (1992) have stated:

> *A central dilemma in child protection work is that getting the label wrong results in severe suffering, whether the situation is investigated under the child protection procedures, possibly involving the removal of the child, or whether the child is left in an abusive situation . . . these are critical questions of more than stigma and civil liberty; they entail inflicting severe emotional abuse.*

Both social and policy attitudes to child protection have then, even in the recent past, swung between extremes of protecting the child at all costs (with large numbers of children therefore being removed from their families) to supporting the parents and keeping the child within the home, again almost at any cost. Professionals involved in child protection therefore experience considerable uncertainty about their role. They are practising in a high-risk field, both in terms of the effects on children and families of their actions (or failure to act) and the likelihood of blame if they are perceived to fail.

THE HEALTH PROFESSIONALS INVOLVED

The health professionals who have most involvement in child protection are health visitors, paediatricians and child and adolescent mental health specialists, including psychiatrists and psychologists. School nurses have also developed an increasing role in child protection in recent years. For all these individuals, although there will be involvement with parents and carers, the child is clearly the focus of their attention and actions. However, considerable difficulties may arise for health professionals who have an alleged abuser as their patient or client. This is a particular problem for those who work in adult mental health services and for general medical practitioners. There are ethical tensions when the interests of the parent/carer clash with those of the child—in particular, when this challenges the assumption that parents are caring and collaborative in the medical treatment of their children (White *et al.*, 1982).

Health visitors

Health visitors are likely to have the most contact with infants and their families. They have been criticised in Part 8 Reviews[1] into deaths or serious injury of children for their failure both to recognise abuse and to act when it has been recognised. Health visitors are in a uniquely difficult situation. They are line managed through a nursing hierarchy responsible to the health care provider management but, in terms of dealing with patients they have historically been expected to seek advice or discuss the issues with the general medical practitioner (family doctor) whose practice population they cover. This can cause further conflict: in recent

---

[1] Case reviews are described in Part 8 of *Working Together*, hence "Part 8 Reviews". They are conducted by individual agencies, and an overview report produced by the local Area Child Protection Committee, when a child dies (where child abuse is confirmed or suspected) or when a child protection issue likely to be of major public concern arises.

years, health visitors have been increasingly expected to act to safeguard children, even, when necessary, going against the views of the general practitioner. For some health visitors this has been a liberation, but clearly for many it has created considerable role conflict.

Paediatricians

Recent years have seen increasing specialisation in child protection for both doctors and nurses. The role of paediatricians in the diagnosis of child sexual abuse was highlighted by the Cleveland Inquiry: although it criticised some of the actions of the paediatricians involved, there was also understanding of the difficulties in the diagnosis and management of child sexual abuse. The report stated:

> It is difficult for professionals to balance the conflicting interests and needs in the enormously important and delicate field of child sexual abuse. We hope that professionals will not as a result of the Cleveland experience stand back and hesitate to act to protect the children.

This summarises the problem for all those involved in child protection but particularly for those who are expected to make a "diagnosis". The signs of actual physical abuse may be less open to argument, but in sexual abuse, emotional abuse and neglect, signs may be difficult to interpret and issues may rest on professional opinion. This is an area which is frequently challenged in Court and the Court experience is a clear source of stress. Senior nurses and paediatricians given the responsibility for providing expert advice on child protection matters and working with other agencies to develop policy and procedures, training and monitoring (the designated professionals) are unlikely to have any colleagues with equivalent experience or expertise within their area and may experience considerable professional isolation.

General practitioners

General practitioners are often in the situation of knowing the parent or carer before any allegation of abuse is made, and indeed may have cared for the family across several generations. They have been criticised in Part 8 Reviews for failure to recognise abuse, failure to refer to social services and failure to assist with ongoing assessment. Lack of attendance by the general practitioner at case conferences[2] is an almost universal criticism

---

[2] *Working Together* states that the child protection conference is "the prime forum for sharing information and concerns, analysing risk and recommending responsibility for action".

in Part 8 Reviews which involve them. Work with a focus group of general practitioners by the first author revealed many concerns. For example, they were unhappy about sharing with social workers medical information on alleged abusers and the wider family and described low confidence in the other agencies' abilities to protect children and maintain confidentiality. These perceptions of other agencies cause not only stress for the general practitioner but also for other health professionals (in particular, health visitors) working with them. They may be working effectively with colleagues in social services but feel "blocked" by the general practitioner's attitude.

Adult mental health professionals

These professionals have been particularly criticised for failure to communicate with other health care professionals and other agencies since they often appear reluctant to share suspicions or knowledge about their client's abusive acts. In his study of 100 Part 8 Reviews, Falkov (1996) found ". . . there was little emphasis on child protection and on the nature of children's experiences prior to their premature deaths amongst adult (mental health) services".

Issues around confidentiality are real and can cause considerable conflict between health care professionals and between agencies. In one case, a senior nurse in child protection experienced considerable difficulty in acting to protect a child when an adult mental health professional refused to name a parent who was known be placing an infant at risk of serious harm.

SOURCES AND LEVELS OF STRESS

It is clear from this description of roles that those involved in child protection face very difficult conflicts at every level of their work and often have inadequate support. In addition, they are potentially subject to considerable external scrutiny, more so than other workers. They are often criticised in Part 8 Review reports, and being involved in a case leading to a review can cause considerable distress. Moreover, the designated professionals in each area are usually responsible for conducting the part of the review relating to the health service (unless directly involved in the case), thus adding to their workload. As management of cases of suspected child abuse becomes more complex, with an increasing need for detailed assessment and the knowledge that indecision or decisions made are likely to be criticised, many senior doctors and nurses in child protection find themselves unable to cope with increasing work demands. Finally, the need to appear in Court, with the questioning of one's opinions and practice and the disruption of normal work schedules, is a particular stress.

There are also examples of particular types of abuse or abusive situations which can cause considerable conflict between health professionals. Induced illness syndrome or Munchausen syndrome by proxy occurs when a parent or carer (most often female) (Rosenberg, 1987) repeatedly injures her child in order to attract medical attention. For example, in a case known to the first author, a child underwent multiple unnecessary operations. Initial concerns of school nurses provoked angry reactions from paediatric surgeons and others. Considerable distress was caused to many health care professionals before the child was finally protected and the perpetrator charged and found guilty. In this case it was many months after the initial concern that action was taken, and the child continued to be injured over this period.

Child protection clearly places considerable emotional demands on health care professionals, and these may be exacerbated further by an interaction with their individual experiences. West (1997) has described three main issues in this regard. First, the adult's revulsion about what has happened to children, in particular when dealing with more extreme forms of abuse such as paedophile rings and other forms of ritual abuse; second, the issues relating to the professionals themselves in terms of their own past experience of childhood and family life; and third, the issues of counter-transference. The professional may develop feelings of violation and powerlessness, guilt and sadness: Youngson (1993) conducted a survey of professionals working with ritually abused people and found that, of 71 respondents, 97% had negative changes in emotional and physical health, 50% of those in partnerships had difficulties in their relationships, and 38% experienced sexual problems.

On top of these potential stressors particular to child protection, come all the organisational difficulties including professional isolation, role ambiguity and constraints. Although not specific to health care professionals involved in child protection, these difficulties may be more pronounced due to the high public profile and oscillating social and policy attitudes to child protection described previously.

Although the difficulties appear clear, no study has been carried out to see what issues are actually seen as stressors, or what levels of psychological symptoms exist in senior health professionals working in child protection. Before this is done interventions on their behalf will undoubtedly fail. With a view to productive changes, we therefore set up a study to find their levels and sources of stress and their views on what changes and intervention might help.

THE CHILD PROTECTION DESIGNATED PROFESSIONALS STUDY

In September 1996, a questionnaire was sent to all designated child protection doctors and nurses in the northern and Yorkshire region of Britain. This contained demographic questions, stress and depression assessments, the Sources of Stress Questionnaire (SSQ) concerning the levels and frequencies of various potential stressors, and an open-ended question about how their jobs could be improved. The 27 (64%) returned consisted of 10 nurses and 17 doctors with a range of years within child protection from 2 years to 20.

Stress and depression levels

Stress was measured using the 12-item version of the General Health Questionnaire (GHQ; Goldberg, 1972) and depression by using the item mean of the depression scale of the Symptom Check-List-90 (SCL-90; Derogatis *et al.*, 1973) with the threshold of 1.5 or above used to signify above threshold levels of depression (Firth-Cozens, 1987).

In terms of general stress, there were seven (26%) scoring at the conservative threshold of 4 or above and 12 (44%) scoring at 3 or above. This is considerably higher than population studies—for example, the British Household Panel Survey for 1993 showed overall levels of 18% for the working population using the more stringent threshold—but similar to the proportion of 27% found in health professionals as a whole (Wall *et al.*, 1997).

In terms of depression, there were six (22%) scoring at or above the threshold of 1.5 (though one left this scale unanswered after scoring very high on the GHQ). This is again higher than community norms and other health worker studies; for example, a recent study of general practitioners showed 18% above threshold using the same instrument (Firth-Cozens, 1997). There were no significant differences in levels of depression or stress between nurses and doctors.

In terms of objective work factors, the more years respondents had spent in child protection the higher their stress levels ($r=0.25$), but not significantly so; nor were any of the other work variables related significantly to either stress or depression, apart from the proportion of time spent in child protection which was highly related to both ($r=0.62$, $p<0.01$).

The sources of stress

Table 10.1 sets out the sources of stress from the SSQ in terms of the mean perceived levels and frequencies of each job-related item. It can be seen that the highest levels of stress are seen as caused by the fear of making mistakes, followed by overwork and organisational change, and these are the main stressors for both nurses and paediatricians. Although stress caused by work relationships was relatively frequent, it did not cause high levels of stress. Doctors found the most difficult group to relate to were fellow paediatricians followed by senior managers, while nurses found social services personnel followed by senior managers their most difficult groups. The most frequent stressor is overwork, followed by relationships with paediatric colleagues and organisational change.

Table 10.1:   Levels and frequencies of perceived stressors and relationship of levels to SCL depression scores

Stressor	Level of stress Mean (sd)	Frequency Mean (sd)	Relationship with depression
Making mistakes	2.5 (1.4)	1.1 (0.3)	0.24
Overwork	2.4 (1.0)	1.8 (0.4)	0.66‡
Organisational change	2.0 (0.9)	1.6 (0.5)	0.33
Effects of job on personal life	2.0 (1.2)	1.5 (0.7)	0.68‡
Conflicts between career and personal life	1.7 (1.3)	1.1 (0.7)	0.57
Talking to distressed relatives	1.4 (1.0)	1.1 (0.7)	−0.14
Having too much responsibility	1.4 (1.3)	0.9 (0.7)	0.38
Dealing with parents	1.4 (1.1)	1.1 (0.8)	0.27
Senior managers in Trusts	1.2 (0.9)	0.9 (0.6)	0.41*
Fear of litigation	1.1 (1.1)	0.7 (0.6)	0.29
Paediatric colleagues	1.1 (1.1)	1.6 (0.6)	0.37
Threat of violence	1.1 (1.1)	0.7 (0.7)	0.03
General practitioners	1.0 (0.9)	1.2 (0.7)	0.33
Social services	1.0 (0.8)	1.4 (0.7)	0.28
Making decisions	0.9 (0.9)	1.4 (0.8)	0.32
Nursing colleagues	0.9 (1.0)	1.4 (0.8)	0.19
Child and adolescent mental health professionals	0.9 (1.0)	1.1 (0.8)	0.27
Adult mental health professionals	0.9 (1.2)	0.7 (0.6)	0.42
Dealing with children	0.7 (0.7)	1.1 (0.8)	0.56†
Dealing with police	0.6 (0.7)	1.1 (0.7)	0.37

* $p < 0.5$;   † $p < 0.1$;   ‡ $p < 0.001$

The relationship of each SSQ item to the depression score is set out in the final column. (Stress scores behave in similar ways.) This shows that there are significant correlations between depression levels and levels of stress caused by overwork, effects of job on personal life, conflicts between career and personal life (both of which are likely to be a reflection of overwork), relationships with senior managers in Trusts and with adult mental health professionals, as well as the stress caused by dealings with children. However, we are unable to comment on the direction of causation; it may be that overwork is actually causing the high depression levels, or it may be that those who are suffering from depression become more sensitised to the workload and to difficulties in relationships.

Respondents were also asked to write about a stressful event which had happened to them within the past month. These qualitative accounts provide more detailed information on areas which might not have been listed in the SSQ reported above. The 21 accounts provided fell into six categories: The nature of the work (7 accounts); overwork/too few resources (5); court appearances (3); poor management (2); failure of groups to work together for child's benefit (2); staff ineptitude or lack of training (1); and administrative tasks and bureaucracy (1). The largest category, involving the nature of the work itself, included accounts of dealings with aggressive parents, having doubts about the existence of abuse, making decisions without full knowledge, and watching children suffer through indecision, etc.

Respondents were also asked to rate the degree of stress in the incident they described on a scale of 1 (slightly stressful) to 4 (extremely stressful). The category of incidents which created the most stress was court appearances (3.3); followed by the failure of groups such as social services and mental health to work together (3.0); overload (2.8); and poor management (2.7). The largest category, the nature of the work, had one of the lowest stress scores (2.3).

With such small numbers in the categories, differences in perceived stressfulness may be largely due to the individual respondent, rather than to any real differences between the effects of particular stressors. Having made that caveat, the varying levels may indicate that it is aspects of the job which staff see as able to be changed but which continue to exist—a manager's lack of appreciation, the inability to get a room to interview parents, the Courtroom attack, the failure of people to work together competently for the child's benefit—that are actually the most problematic, rather than the intrinsically difficult nature of the job itself. The earlier finding—that there is a strong relationship between the proportion of time spent in child protection work and stress, as well as a nonsignificant relationship between the number of years involved in the work and stress—would suggest evidence of burnout (see Chapter 2), but may be as much about having to deal with these "unnecessary" problems year after year as it is with the doubts and difficulties of the work itself. This, of course, is important in terms of bringing about change.

WHAT CAN BE DONE TO IMPROVE THE WORK?

Suggestions on ways to change working practice for the better come both from the survey and from the workshop of child protection professionals held with the authors to discuss the results. They fall into the following categories:

- The need for extra resources
- Courts
- Supervision, training and time out
- The multi-agency service
- Role issues
- Genuine child protection

The need for extra resources

The largest group concerned the need for increased resources, reflecting one of the main stressors. One respondent stated: "Nothing more in the way of help is ever offered until there is a disastrous crisis". Another wrote: "I get exasperated by a government that enacts good legislation (the 1989 Children Act) and then fails to resource it." Particular suggestions for change in this area are:

> We need to work with the fact that we are counter to the current culture of managed care. . . . We cannot meaningfully count up episodes in the usual way, our outcomes are not so clear-cut as others' may be, and we have to cope with greater publicity being given to failures than to success. In addition, this is a service which represents an aspect of our society that most people would rather deny existed, so it is always tempting for others to overlook what we need to do the job better.

> We need to be clearer about how we use our time and what our outcomes are. Outcome measurement itself should be as wide as possible so that the full impact on members of the family and community is more apparent. This should make us more clearly useful to purchasers.

> At times CP work is very busy. A single complex case can take up all one's time and other work has to be shelved or done at night and weekends. I should like to have a contract which allows payment for this excess work which can crop up at any time.

Courts

The need to have courts change in the way they operate in terms of the enormous time-wasting caused to both child protection workers and the court itself was emphasised along with the emotional difficulties faced by having to be a witness. Suggestions included:

> *Persuade the legal system to review the way it organises cases and "demands" our time and treats us without due regard to our other responsibilities.*
>
> *We need to **acquire more individual control** so that the experience is not so stressful. This might be enhanced by:*

- *Training*
  - *In assertion (to say no, assert our rights, etc.)*
  - *Along with local authority so that both can understand the issues.*
  - *For report-writing since this can make a large difference in reducing the numbers of court appearances.*
  - *In court appearances.*

- ***Clarify your role and the full extent of your expertise.***
- ***Where two parents are involved, go for a subpoena.***

> *A **local Court User Group** works well. This consists of magistrates, family court members, social services, solicitors, etc. It provides a forum for clarifying roles and expertise and for understanding each others' points of view and issues. It can bring about change (e.g. reducing time-wasting, waiting areas, etc.). If there is difficulty in setting one up locally, then at least organise or attend one-off meetings to address the issues involved.*
>
> ***Campaign for larger change,*** *for example, to have "medical evidence" as "neutral" given by recognised experts to cut out the so-called experts whose aim is to fudge the evidence so the case is dropped.*

Supervision, training and time out

Supervision is usually received on an ad hoc footing; for example, from local clinical psychologists, with the police or social services. There should be a contract with the purchasers which makes regular supervision part of the job. Most people saw this type of counselling supervision (at least fortnightly) as externally provided and paid for within the contract. There is also a need for occasional specialist or technical supervision; e.g. from forensic expert, orthopaedic experts, etc. Other suggestions included:

[Despite having good colleagues and good relationships with social service and child psychiatry] I would benefit from time to time from some external and independent supervision from an expert. The problem is that the experts are too busy to take on such a task.

There should be an obligatory "time out" (e.g. three months in two years) for front-line child protection workers.

The level of work is manageable for me, but the emotional effect is one I have difficulty acknowledging. Perhaps some regular "debriefs" or "mental health" time in the way of extra holidays, time outs, sabbaticals, etc. I now have a General Manager who recognises the need for this—if she can, why can't other managers?

One respondent also wrote of the need to research, reflect upon and review the service:

The amount of day-to-day work does not allow time for any research or development. We also need to continually review service and practice across all agencies, especially in one's own agency. Reviewing the work at yearly time-outs would be very useful.

The multi-agency service

Respondents who suggested a multi-agency child protection service wrote in response to stressful incidents such as: "The inability to get Social Services and mental health to work together for the benefit of a child. Each service was claiming the other was responsible and the child received no service at all. The health visitor who is not a gateway to services was left trying to sort it out." Suggestions for change included:

Child protection may be less stressful, more efficient and more cohesive in standards if all workers work from a centralised site and have opportunities to see one another, intermingle disciplines and obtain a more sensible perspective. Patch-based work makes fragmentation, loneliness and maverick behaviour far more likely. It is also much more expensive.

Work as a multi-agency, multidisciplinary Child Protection Team: sharing resources (offices, clerical staff, etc.), budget, and ideas.

Role issues

One respondent wanted the child-protection role to be completely full time. However, given the fact that stress levels seem to rise as the CP proportion increases, this may not be a good idea unless and until other aspects of the work are improved. Increased role clarity is often associated with a lowering of stress levels (Warr, 1987) and this is likely to be particularly helpful in a job where uncertainty in many of its key aspects is so paramount. One respondent wrote: "The standard 'No child will die' is unrealistic and makes failure inevitable. We need clearer standards about what we can do, what is possible, etc."

Genuine child protection

There were some who would like to see the whole strategic direction of endeavour turned around to encourage genuine child protection rather than what they saw as largely rescue. For example:

There is an urgent need for services to support families in their child-rearing. There should be more joint initiatives between social services, health, education, community development and volunteers.

We must separate the health needs of the child from the ability of the parent to organise it. Children are crossed off the lists of GPs, speech therapists, child psychologists, etc., simply because their parents are too lazy, stupid or simply unable to organise a clinic visit. The child's needs must come first.

Go for focused projects in small areas. This makes success more likely which is good for individual morale as well as the community involved. The larger politics involved can be tackled through professional groups and charities. Newcastle has a multidisciplinary project on prevention taking place, financed by charities.

We need to champion the roles of health visitors as there are risks that they may be vanishing and then resurrected. There should be an initiative to look at their work, roles and training in detail.

Health visitors' prioritising for high dependency is useful. It allows you to target the at-risk families. The rest (30%) who do not show obvious risk factors are a population that needs further research.

We should also be protecting, not rescuing, the staff.

ACKNOWLEDGEMENTS

The coding, data entry and initial analyses of the questionnaires were carried out by Rob Firth in the Psychology Department, University of Leeds.

REFERENCES

Cm 412 (1988). Report of the Inquiry into Child Abuse in Cleveland 1987. London: HMSO.

De Mause, L. (1976). The evolution of childhood. In L. de Mause (Ed.) *The History of Child Relationships as a Factor in History*. London: Souvenir Press.

Derogatis, L.R., Lipman, R.S. and Covi, M.D. (1973). SCL-90: an outpatient psychiatric rating scale—preliminary report. *Psychopharmacology Bulletin*, **9**, 13–20.

Donaldson, L.J. and O'Brien, S.J. (1995). Press coverage of the Cleveland Child Sexual Abuse Inquiry: a source of public enlightenment? *Journal of Public Health Medicine*, **17**, 70–76

Falkov, A. (1996). *Fatal Abuse and Parental Psychiatric Disorders*. An analysis of 100 Area Child Protection Committee Case Reviews conducted under the terms of Part 8 of *Working Together Under the Children Act 1989*. London: Department of Health.

Firth-Cozens, J. (1987). Emotional distress in junior house officers. *British Medical Journal*, **295**, 533–536.

Firth-Cozens, J. (1997). Predicting stress in general practitioners: 10 year follow up postal survey. *British Medical Journal*, **315**, 34–35.

Goldberg, D.P. (1972). *The Detection of Psychiatric Illness by Questionnaire. Maudsley Monograph No. 21*. London: Oxford University Press.

Hallet, C. and Birchall, E. (1992). *Coordination and Child Protection: A Review of the Literature* (p. 117). London: HMSO.

Home Office, Department of Health, Welsh Office (1991). *Working Together Under the Children Act 1989*. London: HMSO.

Kempe, C.H. and Helfer, R. (1972). *Helping the Battered Child and his Family*. Philadelphia: Lippincott.

Mollon, P. (1988). Oedipus now: the psychoanalytic approach to trauma and child abuse. *Changes*, **6**, 17–19.

Reder, P., Duncan, S. and Gray, M. (1993). *Beyond Blame. Child Abuse Tragedies Revisited*. London: Routledge.

Rosenberg, D. (1987). Web of deceit: a literature review of Munchausen Syndrome by proxy. *Child Abuse and Neglect*, **11**, 547–563.

Wall, T.D., Bolden, R.I., Borrill, C.S., Carter, A.J., Golya, D.A., Hardy, G.E., Haynes, C.E., Rick, J.E., Shapiro, D. and West, M. (1997). Minor psychiatric disorder in NHS trust staff: occupational and gender differences. *British Journal of Psychiatry*, **171**, 519–523.

Warr, P. (1987). *Work, Unemployment and Mental Health*, Oxford: Oxford University Press.

White, E.R., Guehl, R.L., White, A.H., Spoltswood, J.P. and Morgenstern, M.S. (1982). Current concepts of child abuse and neglect. *Journal of Legal Medicine*, 41–57.

Youngson, S.C. (1993). Ritual abuse: consequences for professionals. *Child Abuse Review*, **2**, 251–262.

PART III

INTERVENTIONS FOR STRESS

11

ORGANISATIONAL INTERVENTIONS TO REDUCE STRESS IN HEALTH CARE PROFESSIONALS

Lawrence R. Murphy

INTRODUCTION

Although previous chapters in this book described the stressful nature of health care work, two issues bear repeating. First, health care professions have always been identified as high-stress occupations (e.g. Payne and Firth-Cozens, 1987), owing to a combination of psychosocial factors (high workload, role conflict/ambiguity, low autonomy), rotating shift work, and exposure to infectious, hazardous and physical agents. Second, massive restructuring in the health care industry during the past decade has further increased job stress and associated health consequences because many restructuring efforts have not paid sufficient attention to fundamental principles of organisation development and change (Pindus and Greiner, 1997; Short, 1997). The result has been restructured work systems designed to address management needs (e.g. reduced inefficiency and cost containment), but which largely ignored the human element. It is not surprising that the US Advisory Commission on the Health Care

Stress in Health Professionals. Edited by Jenny Firth-Cozens and Roy L. Payne
© 1999 John Wiley & Sons Ltd

Industry recently recommended that health care organisations ". . . address the serious morale problems that exist among health care workers in many sectors of the industry" (President's Advisory Commission on Consumer Protection and Quality in the Health Care Industry, 1998).

This chapter deals with organisational interventions to reduce stress and improve the quality of work life for health care professionals, and is organised around two fundamental questions: First, what types of intervention have been successful in reducing stress in health care settings? Second: What are the key features or ingredients of successful interventions? The first part of the chapter describes successful interventions in health care settings, with special reference to studies published in the past five years (i.e. 1994–1998). The second part lists core elements of successful stress interventions which have been extracted from published studies.

WHAT ARE ORGANISATIONAL STRESS INTERVENTIONS?

Organisational stress interventions are defined as actions to eliminate or reduce stressful job characteristics and working conditions to improve worker well-being. In medical terminology, such interventions would be classified as primary prevention because they seek to remove or reduce the sources of stress at work (e.g. clarifying role relationships, increasing autonomy, reducing excessive workload). Secondary prevention (e.g. helping workers reduce stress symptoms by improving coping skills), and tertiary prevention (e.g., treating workers with stress-related disorders via medical or employee assistance programmes) are not reviewed here. For descriptions of secondary and tertiary stress prevention studies, see Murphy (1996) and Berridge *et al.* (1997).

EXAMPLES OF SUCCESSFUL STRESS INTERVENTIONS IN HEALTH CARE SETTINGS

In contrast to the large and increasing literature on job stress, organisational stress intervention studies are far less common. One reason for the scarcity of studies is that intervening to reduce job stress is not an exact science, and universal "prescriptions" are not possible, as they are with stress management programmes (Cooper and Cartwright, 1997; Murphy, 1996). This is especially true in health care settings because of the number and diversity of health-related occupations. Another reason is that organisational interventions are difficult to implement in work settings, often requiring substantial disruptions in work schedules and routines which management will not sanction.

Nevertheless, a number of studies were found which evaluated organisational interventions in health care settings, and reported positive post-intervention effects. Five types of intervention are described, each taking a different approach to stress prevention. Most studies focused on providing health care workers with greater input into decision making, and a few studies had a broader focus than simply reducing worker stress (e.g. improving efficiency and reducing costs). Taken together, these case studies provide an indication of the variety of stress interventions being tested in health care settings.

A multi-component intervention

The St Paul Fire and Marine Insurance Company evaluated the impact of a multi-component stress intervention on the frequency of medication errors and medical malpractice claims (Jones et al., 1988). The authors first demonstrated that there was a statistically significant association between levels of job stress and medication errors and malpractice claims. Next, they designed an intervention consisting of multiple activities:

- communicating the results of an employee stress survey to top management and all employees;
- small group sessions with top management to obtain employee input on sources of stress at work and ways to reduce stress;
- policy and procedural changes aimed at improving communication;
- education of employees about the nature and sources of stress at work;
- establishment of an employee assistance programme for employees and their families.

In one study, the frequency of medication errors was reduced by 50% after the intervention was installed in a 700-bed hospital. In a second study, the authors found that malpractice claims were 70% lower in a group of 22 hospitals which implemented stress management activities than a matched group of 22 control hospitals.

The problem with multi-component interventions is that it is impossible to tease out the relative effectiveness of individual features of the intervention. On the other hand, broad-based interventions suggest greater commitment by management (provision of more programmes, more resources, etc.), which in turn implies a more supportive culture. The extent to which these implications are true, and actually contributed to the success of the interventions, is unknown. However, a good deal of research suggests that contextual factors, such as management commitment and a supportive work environment, are vital aspects of successful organisational interventions in health care settings (e.g. Jones et al., 1997).

Innovative coping

A series of articles by West (1989) and Bunce and West (1994, 1996) investigated the frequency and effectiveness of innovative coping as a means of reducing job stress. Innovative coping refers to new strategies or tactics devised and applied by workers as a means of reducing excessive demands at work. In an early study of innovative coping, West (1989) found that innovation among health care workers tends to occur when workload and supervisory support are high. Most of the innovations which were implemented dealt with changes in objectives, working methods, relationships and new skill development. Later studies confirmed the use of innovative coping by health care workers as a stress-reduction strategy, and also described how innovative coping fits into major models of job stress and health, such as person–environment (P–E) fit and demand/control models (Bunce and West, 1994, 1996).

Of course, innovative coping can only be effective if workers have the discretion and authority to implement changes. The health care workers in the studies mentioned above had a high level of discretion, along with high workload. In terms of Karasek's demand–control model, the combination of high demands + high control would place the workers into the "active" cell of the 2×2 matrix, which should be associated with stimulation, growth and low strain (Karasek, 1979).

Work redesign

Three studies are described, two of which used worker participatory methods, and all three tested the work redesign on a pilot basis. The first was reported by Murphy et al. (1994) and involved redesign of a hospital in a rural location. The impetus for change were role conflicts in the care delivery system and frustration at prior attempts to institute change. A worker participation process was used to develop a new patient-care delivery model because staff participation and worker ownership of the new model were considered crucial to success. A team was formed with representatives from each nursing skill level and work shift. Through weekly meetings, and using continuous process improvement tools, the team analysed the current patient care delivery system to identify weaknesses and generate ideas for improvement. A workload measurement assessment also was performed and the results integrated into the work redesign process. An outside consultant was used to facilitate the entire redesign process.

The redesigned patient care delivery system consisted of teams, each responsible for 10–12 patients. Each team consisted of a registered nurse team leader, a licensed practical nurse care giver, unit service assistants and unit-based clerical support staff. The unit service assistant was a new job category responsible for transportation, patient comfort, activities of daily living, vital signs, and intake/output. Also, working arrangements were consolidated into two 12-hour shifts. The new model was implemented on one unit of the hospital as a pilot study. Results indicated a significant improvement in worker satisfaction, and reports from nursing staff indicated reduced stress, improved co-operation between shifts, and less wasted time at work. Turnover was reduced by 11% and unplanned single-day absenteeism dropped by 66%. Staff participation in decision-making, commitment by top management, and "buy-in" of nursing management were identified as the key factors contributing to the success of the redesign effort.

A second study (Abts *et al.*, 1994) involved a 50-bed surgical unit which was facing a large registered nurse vacancy rate and mandatory overtime, plus nurse complaints of stress, frustration and extreme overwork. Acting on advice from a consultant, nursing management initiated a pilot study to redesign the patient care delivery system. A steering committee was formed containing senior managers of nursing, surgical services, pharmacy, nutrition service, staff development, housekeeping, and two staff nurses. The committee identified broad goals for the redesign project and established task forces to analyse work areas to improve patient care and decrease staff workload. A 10-week pilot study was initiated. Redesign changes included a team-based care delivery system consisting of discrete, 16–17 bed care modules, physical environment changes to reduce noise and general activity at the nursing station, and an improved communication system for patient assignments, nursing updates, and bi-weekly module updates. Although the new module patient care delivery system resulted in a decrease of registered nurses in the staff mix, analyses of survey data indicated improvements in both patient and staff satisfaction. Also, job stress levels, which were high before the pilot, were reduced significantly after the 10-week job redesign pilot study.

A third study, conducted in the Netherlands, introduced a new work design called "integrated nursing" into four experimental units of Groningen Hospital (Molleman and Van Knippenberg, 1995). The work redesign did not appear to have substantial involvement of nursing staff, although the staff did participate in the development of a new records system and the redrafting of job descriptions. The new work design involved two elements: patient allocation and nursing process. In the former, nurses were assigned a small number of patients and performed a wide range of services for each one. Nursing process refers to a series of steps that are sequentially accomplished by the nurse (e.g. assess patient needs, formulate care objectives, list specific actions to be taken, etc.). It was assumed that the new design would result in job enlargement and job enrichment, and foster more control for nurses at lower hierarchical levels.

Nurses received training in the new work design, and a staff nurse supported each experimental unit for 8 hours per week. Comparison units were identified in the same hospital plus two units from another hospital. Analyses of pre- and post-work redesign measures indicated small but statistically significant improvements in perceived control among patients and nurses, but not doctors. Unexpectedly, ratings of nurse performance were *lower* on the experimental units compared to control units. In light of the other two job redesign studies reviewed above, it is possible that the lack of employee involvement in the design process contributed to the weak effects reported.

Caregiver support

Heaney *et al.* (1995) developed a Caregiver Support Programme (CSP) to teach direct care staff about the importance of support at work, to educate them about participatory problem-solving approaches to work-related problems, and to provide them with skills for implementing such approaches in work settings. The CSP was developed by a multi-disciplinary team of researchers. The merits of the CSP were evaluated in an experiment among workers at homes for patients with developmental disabilities or mentally illness. A questionnaire measuring attitudes and perceptions towards work, social support, participatory problem solving, and employee well-being was administered one week before training and five weeks after training.

The experimental group consisted of the manager and one direct care staff person from each of 10 group homes, and they received six training sessions over a 9-week period. Training incorporated active learning techniques like modelling, brainstorming and rehearsal of skills, and much of the content of the training was developed by the participants themselves. The authors reported significant post-training effects on perceived social support, group problem solving, job satisfaction and employee mental health. Efforts to get the trainees to train co-workers at their group home failed; only 30% of participants actually taught co-workers their newly learned skills. The authors provided no information as to why more co-worker teaching of skills did not occur.

Worker empowerment through participatory action research (PAR)

In response to high turnover and complaints of low morale and frustration among Australian aboriginal health workers, Hecker (1997) implemented a worker empowerment intervention, using participatory action research (PAR) methods. The aboriginal health worker is the key health care provider and the point of entry into the health care system for aboriginal communities. Aboriginal health workers typically are not accorded very high status in the health care community and often experience role ambiguity/conflict due to differing expectations of their role from their own communities and the non-aboriginal health care staff (i.e. nurses and doctors). PAR was chosen as the intervention method in order to empower the aboriginal health care workers, involving them not only as participants but also as co-researchers. Focus groups and interviews were conducted with aboriginal health workers, community members, and members of a national health council. Three main issues emerged from analyses of the interview and focus group data: (1) low standard of training, (2) lack of skills in English language, and (3) lack of active participation in health service planning and decision making. Many of the recommendations of the aboriginal health workers were implemented by the national health service, including increasing training opportunities and inclusion of health worker representatives at monthly health service meetings, although no data were presented on post-intervention effects.

Other studies

Several organisational intervention studies were not reviewed above because their primary goal was not to reduce worker stress. Nevertheless, they are noteworthy because the interventions have potential for reducing stress. For example, Hanlon (1986) reviewed a number of studies which attempted to reduce hospital costs through increased worker involvement. The involvement activities included quality of work life programmes and quality circles and were designed to foster greater worker input into decision making and job design. Interventions generated from these involvement activities included changes in work practices, job descriptions, work flow and staffing patterns. The most successful programmes occurred in clerical and administrative areas, and laboratory-based departments. Although nearly all of the studies reported positive cost–benefit results, most of the interventions were short-lived (Hanlon, 1986).

Recent work on reducing musculoskeletal injuries via establishing participatory ergonomic teams (Bohr et al., 1997), and reducing occupational exposure to blood-borne pathogens by improving safety climate and establishing total quality involvement teams (Gershon et al., 1995), could also be considered to be stress-reduction actions. It seems clear that by reducing musculoskeletal injuries and worker exposure to HIV/AIDS, perceived stress at work will be lower.

Finally, a good example of a comprehensive restructuring effort is described in detail by Parsons and Murdaugh (1994). A hospital-wide restructuring effort was initiated at University Medical Center at the University of Arizona Health Sciences Center in the early 1990s (Parsons and Murdaugh, 1994). A patient-centred care model was adopted which focused on restructured care delivery, interdisciplinary team management (including high staff involvement), and a corporate culture emphasising excellence. The objectives of the new model were to enhance the quality of patient care and service, address labour shortages by utilising staff more efficiently, promote cost containment, and maintain and enhance the job satisfaction of all health care providers. Analyses of the effects of the new model in four hospital units revealed increases in satisfaction, meaningfulness of work, internal motivation, feedback and task significance (Parsons and Murdaugh, 1994), all of which suggest lower stress.

CORE FEATURES OF SUCCESSFUL ORGANISATIONAL INTERVENTIONS

What can managers do to reduce stress among health care workers? While the studies reviewed above provide ideas for the types of interventions which can reduce stress in health care workers, prescriptive advice cannot be given in the absence of a careful assessment of the sources of stress at work. An accurate assessment of the job conditions and work environment factors which cause stress is a prerequisite for designing effective stress interventions. The assessment of stress need not be a major undertaking, especially in small organisations. Murphy (1995) describes five levels of assessment which vary in terms of their comprehensiveness, ease of use, and requirements for technical expertise. These include: informal discussions with workers; formal group discussions; monitoring of stress indicators; short checklists/questionnaires; and standardised questionnaires.

The ultimate success of any organisational intervention depends on the presence of three key factors which were extracted from the studies described earlier and from reviews of stress interventions in other work settings. These factors should be viewed as necessary and sufficient conditions for successful stress prevention efforts. Often, the most appropriate interventions for any particular health care setting will emerge once these key features are in place and functional.

1. Worker involvement

Worker involvement and participation in decision making has been the topic of a great deal of research over the years, in health care and in many other work settings (e.g. Cotton, 1997; Hanlon, 1986). This body of research clearly suggests that workers desire to be involved in decisions which affect their work, and that worker involvement results in higher job satisfaction, more autonomy, and improved organisational effectiveness.

Two basic elements are needed for worker involvement to be successful. First, workers need to be provided with the opportunity to participate at all stages of the intervention, from planning to evaluation. Second, management needs to delegate authority to workers for the purpose of introducing, managing, and evaluating the effects of organisational change. Worker input into decision-making and the delegation of authority to make changes is necessary because workers have the most detailed knowledge of their jobs and tasks and the best ideas on how to improve work systems. Also, participation facilitates a sense of ownership and "buy-in" by workers which is required for interventions to be sustained over time. In their recent report, the President's Advisory Commission (1998) recommended the involvement and empowerment of all health care employees in efforts to redesign or change the work environment. Worker involvement works best, and produces the most significant benefits, when top management is supportive and when resistance on the part of middle managers is minimal (Fenton-O'Creevy, 1998).

2. Management commitment

Sustained commitment from top management, and buy-in from middle managers, is absolutely critical to successful, long-term organisational interventions. This is perhaps the single most common reason offered for the success (or failure) of organisational interventions. This is true not only for stress interventions, but for all types of workplace interventions. For example, safety professionals have known for over 20 years that safety programmes will fail if there is a lack of strong management commitment to accident reduction (Cohen, 1977). Today, it is difficult to find a safety article that doesn't mention the fundamental need for management commitment to safety. Whether one is talking about organisational interventions targeting safety, quality improvement, repetitive trauma injuries, or workplace violence, management commitment occupies a central position in successful programmes.

What exactly does management commitment mean? Is it merely a matter of issuing policy statements which affirm commitment to stress prevention? Or are specific actions also required which reinforce and validate management commitment? How is it measured? Unfortunately, the research literature is virtually silent on how to measure management commitment, and it is clear that reliable and valid scales need to be developed for this construct. A few attempts to measure management commitment in a safety context have been published (Zohar, 1980; DeJoy et al., 1995). In terms of stress interventions, such management commitment scales should measure the extent to which top management demonstrates commitment to preventing stress through its policies, procedures, decisions, and actions, as well as the prominence of stress prevention in strategic planning and overall business strategy.

3. Supportive organisational culture

An organisational culture which promotes, supports, and reinforces stress interventions is required for long-term success and should occur as a by-product of strong management commitment. Organisational culture refers to the shared beliefs and assumptions of workers about "how things are done around here" and operates as a contextual factor influencing day-to-day decisions and behaviours (Jansen and Chandler, 1994; Jones et al., 1997; Schein, 1990). Culture is slow to change, and does so only in response to new management policies and core values, and decisions and actions which reflect commitment to those policies and values. A health-enhancing organisational culture would treat stress intervention not as an isolated "programme," but rather as an integral part of the overall business strategy. It would operate from a strong set of core values and encourage innovation and involvement among all employees.

The importance of organisational culture was highlighted over 10 years ago in studies of "magnet" hospitals (Kramer and Schmalenberg, 1988) and confirmed in more recent studies (Sochalski et al., 1997). Magnet hospitals are those which are well known for excellent nursing care and low patient mortality. Magnet hospitals are characterised by flat organisational structures, nurse participation in institutional decision making, emphasis on staff development, nurse self-scheduling and unit-based staffing. These organisational characteristics foster greater staff autonomy, more control over resources, and better relationships between nurses and physicians than non-magnet hospitals (Aiken and Sloane, 1997).

A BROADER AGENDA

In the past decade, many authors have argued for a broader research agenda, one which embraces the concept of "organisational health" (Cox and Howarth, 1990; Jaffe, 1995; Pfeiffer, 1987; Rosen, 1991; Sauter et al., 1996). Organisational health refers to worker health *plus* organisational effectiveness, and challenges the traditional belief that promoting worker health will incur a net cost in terms of organisational effectiveness.

The US National Institute for Occupational Safety and Health (NIOSH) is using this broader perspective in studies of healthy work organisations. A healthy work organisation is defined as one whose culture/climate and management practices promote employee safety and health *plus* organisational effectiveness and performance. This definition accommodates organisational goals of profitability and competitiveness, and worker goals of job satisfaction and well-being. Analyses of data obtained from a major US manufacturing company identified three characteristics of a healthy work organisation: (1) a *culture* in which workers are personally valued, have authority to take actions to solve problems, and are encouraged to express opinions and become involved in decision-making; (2) management commitment to company *values* which emphasise employee growth and development, integrity and honesty in communication, and workforce diversity; and (3) *management practices* such as active leadership and strategic planning, recognising workers for problem solving and high-quality work, and first-line supervisors helping workers plan their future (Murphy and Lim, 1997; Sauter *et al.*, 1996). These results are being replicated in other work settings, and NIOSH is working in collaboration with the Finnish Institute of Occupational Health and the University of Manchester Institute of Science and Technology to develop and refine cross-cultural models of healthy work organisations.

CONCLUSIONS

Much of the restructuring taking place in the health care industry is a response to an increasingly competitive market place, a perceived need to improve the quality of patient care and patient satisfaction, and to reduce inefficiencies in patient care delivery and operating costs. The outcome of such restructuring has been new patient care delivery models, such as patient-focused care, which have been received in a positive manner by some health care workers, but have resulted in excessive workload, "speed-ups," and deskilling for many others (Pindus and Greiner, 1997). Asking people to do more work, learn new skills, and adjust to an endless stream of restructuring, without increases in pay, is a recipe for stress and dissatisfaction.

In many work-restructuring projects, a key element is conspicuous in its absence: the well-being of the worker. Restructuring often focuses on objective or "hardware" issues, such as length of patient stay, speed of admission process, and length of time waiting for tests and procedures. The health care worker often has little input into the redesigned work, and is left to "fit in" with the new structure as best they can (Jaffe and Scott, 1997).

Results of the largest-ever patient satisfaction survey should cause health care organisations to reconsider their focus on "hardware" issues, and elevate the health care professional to a more prominent position in future restructuring efforts. The survey involved over one million patients at 545 US hospitals and 44 states (Regrut, 1997). The 10 factors which correlated most highly with patient satisfaction were interpersonal factors such as staff sensitivity to the inconvenience that hospitalisation causes, cheerfulness of hospital staff, staff concern for privacy, amount of attention paid to special or personal needs, and the friendliness of nurses. Least important were "hardware" factors, such as length of time waiting in the X-ray department, food quality and getting the food that the patient had ordered from the menu, speed of admission process, and how well the television and radio worked.

These results seem clear: the best way to improve patient satisfaction is to improve the satisfaction and well-being of health care workers, which will lead to more positive relationships with patients and foster more positive interpersonal factors in the work environment. The title of the patient satisfaction survey report is provocative: "One million patients have spoken, who will listen?"

REFERENCES

Abts, D., Hofer, M. and Leafgreen, P.K. (1994). Redefining care delivery: a modular system. *Nursing Management*, **25**, 40–46.

Aiken, L.H. and Sloane, M.N. (1997). The effects of specialization and client differentiation on the status of nurses: the case of AIDS. *Journal of Health and Social Behavior*, **38**, 203–210.

Berridge, J., Cooper, C.L. and Highly-Marchington, C. (1997). *Employee Assistance Programmes and Work Counselling*. Chichester: Wiley.

Bohr, P.C., Evanoff, B.A. and Wolf, L.D. (1997). Implementing participatory ergonomics teams among health care workers. *American Journal of Industrial Medicine*, **32**, 190–196.

Bunce, D. and West, M.A. (1994). Changing work environments: innovative responses to occupational stress. *Work and Stress*, **8**, 319–341.

Bunce, D. and West, M.A. (1996). Stress management and innovation interventions at work. *Human Relations*, **49**, 209–232.

Cohen, A. (1977). Factors in successful occupational safety programs. *Journal of Safety Research*, **9**, 168–178.

Cooper, C.L. and Cartwright, S. (1997). *Managing Workplace Stress*. Thousand Oaks, CA: Sage Publications.

Cotton, J.L. (1997). Does employee involvement work? Yes, sometimes. *Journal of Nursing Care Quality*, **12**, 33–45.

Cox, T. and Howarth, I. (1990). Organizational health, culture, and helping. *Work and Stress*, **4**, 107–110.

DeJoy, D., Murphy, L.R. and Gershon, R. (1995). Safety climate in health care settings. In A.C. Bittner and P.C. Champey (Eds) *Advances in Industrial Ergonomics and Safety VII* (pp. 223–929) London: Taylor & Francis.

Fenton-O'Creevy, M. (1998). Employee involvement and the middle manager: evidence from a survey of organizations. *Journal of Organizational Behavior*, **19**, 67–84.

Gershon, R.M., Murphy, L.R., Felknor, S., Vesley, D. and DeJoy, D. (1995). Compliance with universal precautions among health care workers. *American Journal of Infection Control*, **23**, 225–236.

Hanlon, M.D. (1986). Reducing hospital costs through employee involvement strategies. *National Productivity Review*, **5**, 22–31.

Heaney, C.A., Price, R.H. and Rafferty, J. (1995). The caregiver support program: an intervention to increase employee coping resources and enhance mental health. In L.R. Murphy, J.J. Hurrell, S. Sauter and G. Keita (Eds) *Job Stress Interventions*. Washington, DC: American Psychological Association.

Hecker, R. (1997). Participatory action research as a strategy for empowering Aboriginal health workers. *Australian and New Zealand Journal of Public Health*, **21**, 784–778.

Jaffe, D.T. (1995). The healthy company: research paradigms for personal and organizational health. In S.L. Sauter and L.R. Murphy (Eds) *Organizational Risk Factors for Job Stress*. Washington, DC: American Psychological Association.

Jaffe, D. and Scott, C. (1997). The human side of re-engineering. *Healthcare Forum Journal*, **40**, 14–21.

Jansen, E. and Chandler, G.N. (1994). Innovation and restrictive conformity among hospital employees: individual outcomes and organizational considerations. *Hospital and Health Services Administration*, **39**, 63–80.

Jones, J.W., Barge, B.N., Steffy, B.D., Fay, L.M., Kuntz, L.K. and Wuebker, L.J. (1988). Stress and medical malpractice: organizational risk assessment and intervention. *Journal of Applied Psychology*, **73**, 727–735.

Jones, K.R., DeBaca, V. and Yarbrough, M. (1997). Organizational culture assessment before and after implementing patient-focused care. *Nursing Economics*, **15**, 73–80.

Karasek, R.A. (1979). Job demands, job decision latitude, and mental strain: implications for job redesign. *Administrative Science Quarterly*, **24**, 285–308.

Kramer, M. and Schmalenberg, C. (1988). Magnet hospitals: Part I. Institutions of excellence. *Journal of Nursing Administration*, **18**(1), 13–24.

Molleman, E. and Van Knippenberg, A. (1995). Work redesign and the balance of control within the nursing context. *Human Relations*, **48**, 795–814.

Murphy, L.R. (1995). Occupational stress management: current status and future directions. In C.L. Cooper and D.M. Rousseau (Eds). *Trends in Organizational Behavior*, Vol. 2. Chichester: Wiley.

Murphy, L.R. (1996). Stress management in work settings: a critical review of the research literature. *American Journal of Health Promotion*, **11**, 112–135.

Murphy, L.R. and Lim, S.Y. (1997). Characteristics of healthy work organizations. In P. Seppälä, T. Luopajärvi, C.-H. Nygård and M. Mattila (Eds) *From Experience to Innovation* Vol 1) (pp. 513–515). Helsinki, Finland: Finnish Institute of Occupational Health.

Murphy, R., Pearlman, F., Rea, C. and Papazian-Boyce, L. (1994). Work redesign: a return to the basics. *Nursing Management*, **25**, 37–39.

Parsons, M.L. and Murdaugh, C.L. (1994). *Patient-centered Care: A Model for Restructuring*. Gaithersburg, Maryland: Aspen Publishers.

Payne, R. and Firth-Cozens, J. (1987). *Stress in Health Care Professionals*. Chichester: Wiley.

Pfeiffer, G.J. (1987). Corporate health can improve if firms take an organizational approach. *Occupational Safety and Health*, **86**, 96–99.

Pindus, N.M. and Greiner, A. (1997). *The Effects of Health Care Industry Changes on Health Care Workers and Quality of Patient Care: Summary of Literature and Research*. Contract Report (DOL-J-9-M-5-0048, #17) prepared by The Urban Institute. Washington, DC: US Department of Labor.

President's Advisory Commission (1998). *Quality First: Better Health Care for all Americans*. Washington DC: Advisory Commission on Consumer Protection and Quality in the Health Care Industry.

Regrut, B. (1997). *One Million Patients have Spoken: Who will Listen?* South Bend, Indiana: Press, Ganey Associates.

Rosen, R. (1991). *The Healthy Company*. Los Angeles: Jeremy P. Tarcher.

Sauter, S.L., Lim, S.Y. and Murphy, L.R. (1996). Organizational health: a new paradigm for occupational stress research at NIOSH. *Japanese Journal of Occupational Mental Health*, **4**, 248–254.

Schein, E. (1990). Organizational culture. *American Psychologist*, **45**, 109–119.

Short, J. (1997). Psychological effects of stress from restructuring and reorganization. *AAOHN Journal*, **45**, 597–604.

Sochalski, J., Aiken, L.H. and Fagin, C.M. (1997). Hospital restructuring in the United States, Canada, and Western Europe: an outcomes research agenda. *Medical Care*, **35**(10), Special Supplement, OS13-OS25.

West, M.A. (1989). Innovation amongst health care workers. *Social Behavior*, **4**, 173–189.

Zohar, D. (1980). Safety climate in industrial organizations. Theoretical and applied implications. *Journal of Applied Psychology*, **65**, 96–102.

12

STRESS AND INTERVENTIONS FOR STRESS IN GENERAL PRACTITIONERS

John Howie and Mike Porter

INTRODUCTION

> *Nearly all UK general practitioners are self-employed. The "businesses" they operate require to generate their livelihood and management costs, and their principal activity is caring for the patients for whom they contract to provide "general medical services" on behalf of the National Health Service. Between 1990 and 1998, some practices took the opportunity to administer ear-marked NHS funds to purchase a range of secondary care services from "providers" (mainly hospitals) on behalf of their patients; these practices or doctors were described as "fund-holders".*

The first edition of this chapter was written in 1986 at a time when interest in stress in general practitioners (GPs) was just beginning to stimulate research into the topic. This new chapter begins with a review of research since 1986 and then discusses some local attempts to intervene to reduce stress in general practitioners.

Stress in Health Professionals. Edited by Jenny Firth-Cozens and Roy L. Payne
© 1999 John Wiley & Sons Ltd

The mid-1980s saw the setting up of studies of consultation time and quality of patient care (Morrell *et al.*, 1986; Roland *et al.*, 1986; Calnan and Butler, 1988; Ridsdale *et al.*, 1989). These, together with the studies on stress reviewed below, and a rapid decline in applicants to general practice training following the 1990 GP Contract, led the Royal College of General Practitioners to establish a working group "Revaluing General Practice" (McBride and Metcalfe, 1995) and to appoint two Stress Fellows over two years, 1995–1997. The BMA established a national counselling service, and there was a proliferation of local stress management and occupational health developments (Chambers and Campbell, 1996; Chambers and Maxwell, 1996; Sims, 1997).

RESEARCH ON STRESS IN GENERAL PRACTITIONERS: 1986–1997

Cross-sectional psychometric studies

Most studies of stress in general practitioners (and doctors more generally) have relied on cross-sectional, postal questionnaire, psychometric study designs.

Manchester (UMIST) Studies

Following a pilot study of Greater Manchester GPs in 1986 (Makin *et al.*, 1998), Cooper *et al.* (1989) developed a 33-item job stress questionnaire. This was sent, in November 1987, together with instruments to measure job satisfaction, mental health, and personal and demographic factors, to 4,000 GPs in England, and 1,817 GPs returned usable completed questionnaires—a response rate of 45%. Following the introduction of the 1990 GP Contract, Sutherland and Cooper mailed a similar set of research questionnaires to another national sample of 1,500 GPs in July/August 1990 (Sutherland and Cooper, 1992). Unlike the previous, and subsequent survey, the questionnaire was not anonymous and a reminder was sent. A response rate of 61% was obtained, but no details were given on the characteristics of the respondents added by the reminder, or of their effect on reported stress levels. A third, anonymous, survey of 850 GPs was conducted in February 1993 and a response rate of 45% was obtained (Rout and Rout, 1994).

Assuming that the different sample sizes, response rates and times of year do not invalidate the findings, male GPs consistently reported significantly higher levels of free-floating anxiety than the male population norm, with the highest level reported by the 1990 sample. Male GP depression levels were below the population norm in 1987 but were significantly above the norm in 1990 and 1993. Female GPs reported higher levels of free-floating anxiety and depression than male GPs, but they were consistently lower than, or similar to, their population norms, except for anxiety in the 1990 sample. Job-satisfaction was significantly lower in the 1990 and 1993 samples than in the 1987 sample. Female GPs, and UK qualified doctors, were significantly more satisfied than male and overseas qualified GPs.

The majority of mean job stressor item scores was significantly higher in the 1990 and 1993 samples of GPs than for the 1987 sample. Multiple regression analysis of the 1990 sample data (Sutherland and Cooper, 1993) explained 45% of the variance in job satisfaction, with demands of the job and patients' expectations contributing to 21% of the variance, organisational structure 7%, and social support 6%.

Other psychometric studies

In 1994, Appleton *et al.* used instruments similar to those used by Cooper *et al.* (1989) to survey all 406 GP principals in Leeds Health Authority (response rate with reminder: 70%) (Appleton *et al.*, 1998). There were no associations between job satisfaction and practice characteristics, but there was a significant negative association between job satisfaction and GHQ-12 scores, and GPs' perception that work had recently affected their physical health: more nights spent on-call and less use of deputising services were particularly related to poorer physical health.

Caplan reported the results of a cross-sectional survey of 257 Lincolnshire GPs (response rate: 80%), hospital consultants and health service managers (Caplan, 1994). Of the GPs, 48% scored >5 on the GHQ 28, almost twice as many as would be expected from a "control" group of professional and managerial people using the GHQ-30. GPs also scored highly on the depression scale of the HADS (Zigmond and Snaith, 1983), and 14% were identified as having suicidal thoughts (compared with 5% of a sample of consultants and 1.3% of managers). However, the study provided no analysis by gender, age or other possible factors associated with the GPs' relatively high anxiety and depression scores.

In a study of all 896 GP principals in Staffordshire in June 1994 (response rate 69%), Chambers and Campbell reported no significant differences in HADS scores between male and female GPs (Chambers and Campbell, 1996). GPs who lived alone reported higher mean anxiety scores than those who lived with a spouse or a partner, but there was no difference in depression scores. Single-handed GPs reported higher mean anxiety scores than GPs in group practice, but again there was no difference in depression scores. Average practice list size was not associated with either anxiety or depression. Non-fundholders and recent fundholders reported significantly higher anxiety scores than more established fundholders. GPs who were trainers, or in a training practice, reported significantly lower levels of anxiety and depression than doctors not in a training practice. GPs who were more frequently on call reported higher levels of anxiety and depression, and doctors who did not have a half-day were more likely to report higher depression scores.

Finally, the Maslach Burnout Inventory has been used as an indicator of stress in two studies: one of all 295 Northamptonshire GPs in March 1993 (Kirwan and Armstrong, 1995) and the other of 1,232 South Australian GPs in 1987 (Winefield and Anstey, 1991). The British study (response rate with reminder: 83%) found that younger GPs reported higher scores on the "depersonalisation of others" subscale than older GPs, and that part-time GPs reported lower scores on the "emotional exhaustion" subscale than full-time GPs. The Australian study (response rate: 78%) identified higher levels of emotional exhaustion and depersonalisation of others in younger GPs. Male GPs scored higher levels of emotional exhaustion, depersonalisation and job dissatisfaction. Female GPs in most age categories were less likely to be frustrated by difficult patients, or to worry about time or money problems.

Various qualitative studies have largely confirmed these findings (for example, Myerson, 1992).

Longitudinal psychometric studies

Two longitudinal studies of medical students have recently reported follow-up results of students who have now become GPs. Firth-Cozens has reported the results of her longitudinal study of 302 medical students who were in their fourth undergraduate year in 1983–1984 (Firth-Cozens, 1997, 1998). Of these individuals, 74% responded to a follow-up questionnaire in the winter of 1993–1994, of whom 131 were GPs. Approximately 33% of the GPs scored above the threshold for symptoms of stress using the GHQ-12, which is considerably higher than the general working population. There was no correlation between current stress levels and stress levels 10 years previously, nor with practice size or hours worked in the past week. However, high self-criticism (self-blame) as a student was highly correlated with current stress levels, accounting for 12% of the variance. Firth-Cozens (1998) reports that depression and self-criticism as students, along with current sleep levels, were the main predictors of symptoms of depression in men; whereas sibling rivalry as children and current alcohol use were the main predictors in women. Relationships with senior doctors and with patients were their main reported stressors, followed by making mistakes and conflict of career with personal life.

A longitudinal study of all first-year students at Edinburgh medical school in 1986 has recently been completed by Baldwin *et al.* (1997). Relatively few were established GPs by 1996, but she reports that: overwork, the effects of work on personal life, conflicts between career and personal life, making mistakes, making decisions and talking to distressed relatives were the most frequent/severe stressors reported by those who had become GPs.

Observational studies

There have been two "observational" studies of GPs: a descriptive, observational study over 12 months in 1987–1988 in Lothian (Howie *et al.*, 1993); and a controlled, intervention study of Nottinghamshire GPs also in 1987–1988 (Wilson *et al.*, 1991). Unlike the studies reported above, both studies were interested in the relationship between stress and the process and outcome of consultations, and both used short-term measures of stress.

Our Lothian model of GP stress has gone through a number of developments (Porter *et al.*, 1985, 1987, 1989). Eighty-five volunteer GPs collected data on one day in 15 over the year November 1987 to October 1988. Information was returned on 1,536 weekdays, 1,948 routine surgery sessions and 21,707 surgery consultations. Doctors who were less "patient-centred" (as defined by scores on three attitudinal factors derived from Cockburn *et al.*, 1987) saw patients more quickly, prescribed more frequently and reported lower stress levels than more "patient-centred" doctors (Howie *et al.*, 1992). Shorter consultations were associated with less attention to long-term health problems, psycho-social problems and less health promotion. Lower levels of patient satisfaction and enablement were also reported (Howie *et al.*, 1991). These Scottish findings have been supported by research from The Netherlands (Grol *et al.*, 1985, 1990).

The more "patient-centred" doctors reported higher stress levels when working with appointment times that did not fit their preferred consultation style and consultation length. Running late was stressful because patients were kept waiting, and lateness interfered with their other commitments. Attempting to catch up was stressful because they had to adopt a faster consultation style which they found uncomfortable. Multiple regression analysis confirmed that mismatch between booking rates and consultation rates was the most important factors contributing to stress in more patient-centred doctors. Work impinging on family commitments contributed to afternoon stress levels, and being on-call at night was associated with higher stress scores in older doctors both in the afternoon prior to being on-call, and in the morning following being on-call.

The Nottingham controlled intervention study confirmed that doctors who wanted to take longer with patients reported lower stress scores (and higher arousal scores) when they worked with longer booking intervals than with shorter intervals (Wilson *et al.*, 1991).

Conclusions

It is clear from this review that conceptual, methodological and analytical differences and inconsistencies both within and between studies make it difficult to be certain about either the trends in levels of GP stress or the factors contributing to and mediating stress. It is to be hoped that the current longitudinal, and any future, studies will address these rather than contribute to the confusion.

However, putting this to one side, it does appear that GPs experienced raised levels of anxiety and depression over the time that the 1990 GP Contract and the NHS reforms were being introduced. While these high levels may subsequently have fallen slightly, there are still many GPs experiencing levels of stress which are detrimental to their own, and their patients', health and well-being.

Pressures associated with seeing patients, practice management and administration, being on-call at night and having a full (family) life appear to contribute significantly to both short-term and longer-term stress levels. Of particular concern is the finding that younger, male, GPs appear to be at particular risk of the job dissatisfaction, emotional exhaustion and depersonalisation of others.

DEVELOPMENTS AND INTERVENTIONS

The period between the first and second edition of this book was dominated by the lead up to and the consequences of the 1990 NHS reforms and the "new" general practice contract. This section of the chapter combines a narrative account of that history with a description of three more recent research and development projects which have been or are being undertaken under the auspices of our department in Edinburgh, and have a direct or indirect relevance to stress in general practice. The section concludes with a description of one further local initiative aimed at helping stressed doctors and their families which parallels other similar initiatives being undertaken elsewhere (Chambers and Maxwell, 1997; Sims, 1997; Young and Spencer, 1996).

Predictable problems

The 1990 reforms and contract eventually materialised rather suddenly at the end of a period of political posturing by professionals and politicians which dated back at least to the Green Paper of 1986. In this, the Government matched its wish to see greater professional commitments to quality of care and to accountability with the need to ensure value-for-money and to involve consumers in choices about their care. The strategies proposed included a shift in the basis of remuneration away from capitation and "basic practice allowance" towards "fees for services" related to activities encapsulated partly in a "good practice allowance". The new general practice contract required a cluster of screening and preventive activities for which there was insufficient scientific evidence of benefit. New administrative work was required to service this work and either doctors had to do this out of clinical time, or employ staff at an element of personal cost. The publication of consumer "contracts" together with growing trends towards litigation and demand (particularly out-of-hours) and the threat (albeit one that rarely materialised) of managerial policing of compliance with "terms and conditions" of contracts fuelled the ambivalence of doctors to their work. "Role conflict", "role ambiguity" and loss of "job decision latitude" together with "responsibility", "increased work load", and "shift working" proved a mix too much for many. For perhaps the majority of general practitioners, the emphasis on holism that training and consensus was encouraging in their clinical practice was compromised by diversion of both time and emotional commitment to other matters.

Apart from column-inches on stress becoming a regular feature of the professional "weeklies", a combination of disillusionment and stress persuaded many doctors to take early retirement. Others decided to leave general practice for other medical employment. As well as the widely publicised falls in recruitment to training schemes and in applications for advertised vacancies, the profession lost a large percentage of its senior workforce. In Scotland in 1985, 731 out of 2,882 (25%) general practitioners were aged between 55 and 65; in 1996, there were only 386 out of 3,394 (11%) (Scottish Advisory Committee on the Medical Workforce, 1998).

Seeking solutions

In the period following the 1990 NHS changes, this department has been involved in three projects directly or indirectly related to general practice stress. These are summarised below.

The Scottish Shadow Fund-holding Project

The first fund-holding evaluation (and the only one supported by government funding) took place from 1991 to 1993 in the north-east of Scotland. Six practice groups involving 49 doctors recorded details of all their consultations during four two-week periods over two years. In addition, we studied their patterns of prescribing and referral, noted the longitudinal care of patients with selected conditions, assessed their attitudes to issues related to the provision of care, and asked about perceptions of gains and costs on a weekly basis throughout a calendar year.

Two sets of results are relevant. First, fund-holding was associated with patients whose problems were of relatively low prevalence but were mainly bio-medical (diabetes and angina, for example) receiving longer time at consultations and scoring higher on enablement (Howie *et al.*, 1995a, b). On the other hand, patients with relatively more common problems, which often included a more complex mix of medical and behavioural issues (dyspepsia, orthopaedic and mental health problems for example), received shorter consultations and reported poorer outcomes.

Second, doctors—and practice managers—reported perceived costs (non-monetary) as being higher than perceived benefits in the earlier stages of fundholding. By the end of the year, "lead" doctors felt benefits to be greater than costs, but managers (for whom costs were particularly high) still saw costs as higher, as did non-lead doctors who saw relatively little benefit in the change of organisational structure throughout our period of observation.

The relevance of this to stress in general practice more widely is partly that fundholding tended to move the emphasis from "holistic" to "bio-medical" practice (creating role conflict and role ambiguity) which was stressful for those whose orientation was more patient-centred. It was also partly because administrative load was increased without evidence of matching benefit, again stressful for the same reasons.

There have, of course, been benefits. Ownership of decision making moved strongly from secondary care to primary care, and some doctors with interests in organisational and managerial activities found new opportunities and challenges.

Supporting practices with special needs

After completing work on the relationship between consultation length, queuing, stress and quality of care (as described above) we began to take that work into practical application. First we piloted a series of practice audits in which we visited practices with appointment system problems to assess their causes. We asked the doctors to note patient flow, appointment availability and consultation length over a two-week period and to measure "patient satisfaction" at the same time. After analysing the results, we provided feedback and a second meeting with the partners to discuss the implications of our findings and help negotiations towards solutions within the partnerships. We suggested a further two-week recording of data once changes had been implemented, but, in the majority of cases, this completion of the audit loop was not undertaken despite our encouragement. In the second study, we were allocated money for one year specifically to support practices asking help to explore stresses within partnerships. We followed the same methodological approach as in the previous study. Although the studies recruited practices in a different way, the outcomes were so similar that it is appropriate to present the results together. Twenty-six practices took part in the two studies. Twenty-two of them included all partners. In four of them only one doctor was involved. The majority of practices worked in more deprived areas and few were enthusiastic about fundholding. Although we used a similar audit framework for each practice, the details of problems and wishes in individual practices differed, and what we collected—both in terms of process and outcome information—differed sufficiently to make aggregation of our numerical date inappropriate. In addition, to maintain confidentiality we have to present our commentary in general rather than particular terms.

On average, practices worked with eight patients booked per hour. However, "extras" were generally added both during and after surgeries, and surgeries normally ran very late—often finishing an hour or more late for a two-hour surgery. Later consultations were frequently short and problematic for doctors (preoccupied with other tasks) and for patients (annoyed by long periods of waiting). In most of the practices that used our services, surgeries were fully booked at the start of the day, making the receptionists' role in handling appointment requests stressful. Doctors were often unhelpful in agreeing to see "extras" or to speak to patients on the phone; most practices had policies, but partners differed in their willingness to implement them.

Doctors were dominated by a belief that workload should be shared equally. There were no policies for recognising the fact that some doctors see more psychological problems than others and need more time for counselling-type styles. Partners often held ill-informed and unhelpful beliefs about each other's policies for recalling patients for follow-up consultations—a common source of conflict when one or more partners are perceived to fill their surgeries with "easy" consultations. In many partnerships there were sharp and undiscussed polarisations about attitudes to patients, with some doctors clearly no longer empathetic to what they perceived as high levels of unnecessary and unreasonable demands, and others taking wholly different views about the effect of social and psychological pressures in a changing society on patients' general well-being. Quite often difficulties were aggravated by (or sometimes caused by) outside commitments of partners (particularly when unnegotiated), by health problems in partners, by issues of study leave and maternity leave, and by holiday absences and out-of-hours rotas. The issues of administration and whether to encompass fundholding were often the eventual precipitants in deciding to ask for outside help.

The aggregate effect of these issues (almost so common in partnerships as to be normal) varied widely from open and determined efforts to negotiate solutions, through denial of the existence of problems, to dysfunction in addressing them. The dysfunction was aggravated by internal relationships in practices, which ranged from isolation through conspiracy to outright feuding. Age and gender polarisations were often apparent, but the issues of consulting style and work orientation seemed to us the more important. Again the stressors of load and responsibility, and of role conflict and ambiguity, and loss of job decision latitude seemed to summarise what we observed.

Collection of data in the practices provided a welcome—and often therapeutic—opportunity for partners to step back and seek an objective base from which to address problems. Nearly everyone was willing to collect some information about their consultations for a period of two weeks, and patients and reception staff also welcomed the chance to contribute to discussions about the organisation of care in their practices.

The findings were remarkably consistent. Few practices had enough scheduled consultations to meet average demand, and few built in slots to accommodate the extras that nearly always are required. Almost half of the doctors consistently ran late, particularly doctors whose average consultations lasted longer. Most practices had fast doctors (average face-to-face time of 6 minutes or less) and most had slow doctors (average face-to-face time of 9 minutes or more). However, nearly all had 7.5 minute appointments. Given that there is an average of 2 minutes "dead-time" per patient in any surgery, the inevitability of lateness (and of stress) becomes obvious. Patients were generally satisfied with consultations, but often critical of practice organisation and of the accessibility of several doctors.

Feedback of this information helped to open up negotiations on improvements and solutions within the practices concerned. Three main sets of outcomes improved many situations. First, practices understood the nature of their problems better and this helped to bring new understanding between individual doctors about their preferred styles of working. Second, systems were able to be improved either to create more availability or to lengthen consultation slots. (In essence, lengthening slots did not add work but rather reduced waiting and lateness.) Reduced recall rates and more use of repeat prescriptions were examples of other ways of improving effective working. Third, five of the 26 practices were helped to identify that their problems arose from fundamental and unnegotiable differences, and arranged to separate.

The most important reality that these support projects confirmed was that structural and contractual changes within the NHS had precipitated many of the stresses we discussed. Within fixed time constraints holistic care can be delivered more effectively with improved consulting skills but, beyond a certain point, more time is required. A choice between investing in administrative activity, fee-generating item-of-service activity, or unpaid listening time is the reality facing individuals and groups at the time of the latest (1998) reforms. It is sometimes hard for individuals to manage the choice; it is nearly always hard for groups.

Out-of-hours care

The third project was an evaluation of a prototype "out-of-hours co-operative" which was developed by a group of 36 doctors in the Midlothian sector of Lothian, the year preceding attempts in 1995 by the NHS to reconfigure arrangements for out-of-hours services nationally through support for the development of large out-of-hours co-operatives (Heaney *et al.*, 1998). Of particular relevance to this chapter were the strongly positive views of the participating doctors. The responses of the doctors immediately *before* and one year *after* the project began demonstrated its benefit in terms of relief of stress and from stressors: 42% before against 22% after responded that work was interfering with family life; 75% before against 24% after said that they felt stressed the day after a night on call; and 39% before against 23% after said they felt stressed generally in the previous 24 hours (Heaney, personal communication).

The new out-of-hours co-operatives are working on a larger scale than the one described above and further work to evaluate such organisations is in hand. The large volume of telephone consultations handled in on-call periods clearly brings stresses of a new kind and the point of greatest benefit to most people (patients as well as doctors) has yet to be defined. Doctors in some outlying areas remain without realistic access to such facilities and for them the stresses of isolation and the consequences of actual 24-hour availability remain unsolved.

An external stress support service

At the same time as Scottish Office funding became available to fund the practice support service described above, funding was also provided to Lothian Local Medical Committee to purchase an external stress consultancy service for Lothian general practitioners and their families. The service (similar to others previously reported in general practice magazines) was widely publicised and accessed by a telephone call to the consultancy service. Immediate support was offered and rapid arrangements made for a series of up to six long counselling sessions with one of a panel of experts (psychiatrists or psychologists) either within the doctors' (or relatives') geographical area or outwith if preferred for reasons of confidentiality. Because of the confidentiality of the process, only administrative information is available. The contract was taken out on the assumption that about 5% ($n = 500$) of doctors or their families would use the service in the first year, and this was the uptake reported. Eighty-seven per cent of contacts were made by doctors and the remainder by spouses or their children. One-third of episodes was concluded after one month, and almost all within six months. The average number of sessions was 5.5.

CONCLUSIONS

Many of the macro-political changes to the NHS since 1990 have resulted in greater demands on GPs, and to more or less control over working practice in primary care, depending on involvement with fundholding and locality purchasing/commissioning. Over the last 10 years, a number of strategies have been developed to tackle some of the organisational stressors and to provide GPs with better support and coping strategies. This chapter, and Sims's review of stress management strategies (Sims, 1997), have demonstrated that there is an urgent need for an integrative, high-quality research programme into stress and interventions for stress in primary care.

REFERENCES

Appleton, K., House, A. and Dowell, A. (1998). A survey of job satisfaction, sources of stress and psychological symptoms among general practitioners in Leeds. *British Journal of General Practice*, **48**, 1039–1063.

Baldwin, P.J., Dodd, M.D. and Wrate, R.W. (1997). Young doctors' health. I. How do working conditions affect attitudes, health and performance? *Social Science and Medicine*, **45**, 35–40.

Calnan, M. and Butler, J.R. (1988). The economy of time in general practice. *Social Science and Medicine*, **26**, 435–441.

Caplan, R.P. (1994). Stress, anxiety and depression in hospital consultants, general practitioners and senior health service managers. *British Medical Journal*, **309**, 1261–1263.

Chambers, R. and Campbell, I. (1996). Anxiety and depression in general practitioners: associations with type of practice, fundholding, gender and other personal characteristics. *Family Practice*, **13**, 170–173.

Chambers, R. and Maxwell, R. (1996). Helping sick doctors. *British Medical Journal*, **312**, 722–723.

Chambers, R. and Maxwell, R. (1997). *Database of Activities and Initiatives in the UK associated with Reducing GPs' Stress or Improving GP's Well-being.* United Kingdom: Royal College of General Practitioners.

Cockburn, J., Killer, D. and Campbell, E. (1987). Measuring general practitioners' attitudes towards medical care. *Family Practice*, **4**, 192–199.

Cooper, C.L., Rout, U. and Faragher, B. (1989). Mental health, job satisfaction, and job stress among general practitioners. *British Medical Journal*, **298**, 366–370.

Firth-Cozens, J. (1997). Predicting stress in general practitioners: 10 year follow up postal survey. *British Medical Journal*, **315**, 34–35.

Firth-Cozens, J. (1998) Individual and organisational predictors of depression in general practitioners. *British Journal of General Practice*, 1647–1651.

Grol, R., Mokkink, H., Smits, A., Van Eijk, J., Beek, M., Mesker, P. and Mesker-Niesten, J. (1985). Work satisfaction of general practitioners and the quality of patient care. Family Practice, **2**, 128–135.

Grol, R., De Maeseneer, J., Whitfield, M. and Mokkink, H. (1990). Disease-centred versus patient-centred attitudes: comparison of general practitioners in Belgium, Britain and The Netherlands. Family Practice, **7**, 100–103.

Heaney, D., Gorman, D. and Porter, A.M.D. (1998). Self-recorded stress levels for general practitioners before and after forming an out-of-hours primary care centre. *British Journal of General Practice*, **48**, 1077–1078.

Howie, J.G.R., Heaney, D. and Maxwell, M. (1995). Care of patients with selected health problems in fundholding practices in Scotland in 1990 and 1992: needs, process and outcome. *British Journal of General Practice*, **45**, 121–126.

Howie, J.G.R., Heaney, D.J. and Maxwell, M. (1995). *General Practice Fundholding: Shadow Project—An Evaluation* (pp. 1–50). Edinburgh: The University of Edinburgh.

Howie, J.G.R., Hopton, J.L., Heaney, D.J. and Porter, A.M.D. (1992). Attitudes to medical care, the organization of work, and stress among general practitioners. *British Journal of General Practice*, **42**, 181–185.

Howie, J.G.R., Porter, A.M.D., Heaney, D.J. and Hopton, J.L. (1991). Long to short consultation ratio: a proxy measure of quality of care for general practice. *British Journal of General Practice*, **41**, 48–54.

Howie, J.G.R., Porter, A.M.D. and Heaney, D.J. (1993). General practitioners, work and stress. In D.P. Gray (Ed.) *Occasional Papers of the Royal College of General Practitioners* (pp. 18–29). London: The Royal College of General Practitioners.

Kirwan, M. and Armstrong, D. (1995). Investigation of burnout in a sample of British general practitioners. *British Journal of General Practice*, **45**, 259–260.

Makin, P.J., Rout, U. and Cooper, C.L. (1998). Job satisfaction and occupational stress among general practitioners—a pilot study. *Journal of the Royal College of General Practitioners*, **38**, 303–306.

McBride, M. and Metcalfe, D. (1995). General practitioners' low morale: reasons and solutions. *British Journal of General Practice*, **45**, 227–229.

Morrell, D.C., Evans, M.E., Morris, R.W. and Roland, M. (1986). The "five minute" consultation: effect of time constraint on clinical content and patient satisfaction. *British Medical Journal*, **292**, 870–873.

Myerson, S. (1990). Problems in UK general practice since the new contract (1990), and general practitioners' strategies for dealing with them (1992). *Medical Science Research*, **20**, 461–463.

Porter, A.M.D., Howie, J.G.R. and Levinson, A. (1985). Measurement of stress as it affects the work of the general practitioner. *Family Practice*, **2**, 136–146.

Porter, A.M.D., Howie, J.G.R. and Levinson, A. (1987). Stress and the general practitioner. In R. Payne and J. Firth-Cozens (Eds) *Stress in Health Professionals* (pp. 45-69). Chichester: Wiley.

Porter, A.M.D., Howie, J.G.R. and Levinson, A. (1989). Stress in general medical practitioners of the United Kingdom. In F.J. McGigan, W.E. Sime and J.M. Wallace (Eds) *Stress and Tension Control* (pp. 105–118) London: Plenum.

Ridsdale, L., Carruthers, M., Morris, R. and Ridsdale, J. (1989). Study of the effect of time availability on the consultation. *Journal of the Royal College of General Practitioners*, **39**, 488–491.

Roland, M.O., Bartholomew, J., Courtenay, M.J.F., Morris, R.W. and Morrell, D.C. (1986). The "five minute consutation": effect of time constraint on verbal communication. *British Medical Journal*, **292**, 874–876.

Rout, U. and Rout, J.K. (1994). Job satisfaction, mental health and job stress among general practitioners before and after the New Contract—a comparative study. *Family Practice*, **11**, 300–306.

Scottish Advisory Committee on the Medical Workforce (1998). *Report of the Scottish Advisory Committee on the Medical Workforce—General Practice Sub-Committee*. Edinburgh: The Scottish Office Department of Health.

Sims, J. (1997). The evaluation of stress management strategies in general practice: an evidence-led approach. *British Journal of General Practice*, **47**, 577–582.

Sutherland, V.J. and Cooper, C.L. (1992). Job stress, satisfaction, and mental health among general practitioners before and after introduction of new contract. *British Medical Journal*, **304**, 1544–1548.

Sutherland, V.J. and Cooper, C.L. (1993). Identifying distress among general practitioners: predictors of psychological ill-health and job dissatisfaction. *Social Science and Medicine*, **37**, 575–581.

Wilson, A., McDonald, P., Hayes, L. and Cooney, J. (1991). Longer booking intervals in general practice: effects on doctors' stress and arousal. *British Journal of General Practice*, **41**, 184–187.

Winefield, H.R. and Anstey, T.J. (1991). Job stress in general practice: Practitioner age, sex and attitudes as predictors. *Family Practice*, **8**, 140–144.

Young, G. and Spencer, J. (1996). General practitioners' views about the need for a stress support service. *Family Practice*, **13**, 517–521.

Zigmond, A.S. and Snaith, R.P. (1983). The hospital anxiety and depression scale. *Acta Psychiatrica Scandinavica*, **67**, 361–370.

13

STRESS IN THE NURSING DEPARTMENT: LEARNINGS FROM AN EXECUTIVE TEAM RETREAT

Larry Hirschhorn and Linda May

THE TAVISTOCK APPROACH

This chapter is based on the Tavistock approach to understanding how people experience their work in organisations. There are many strands making up this approach (see, for example, those listed in the references). Here we wish to highlight two of its concepts that we use in this chapter. First, all work in organisations, insofar as it is meaningful, contains some risk and therefore stimulates some anxiety. People find many ways to manage this anxiety. For example, they develop their skills, they seek to clarify what bosses or peers ask them to accomplish, and they find ways to gauge their effectiveness. Indeed, when anxiety is adequately managed, people may convert the experience of risk into a sense of excitement or into the welcomed challenge. But some anxieties are sufficiently systemic that they are shared by everyone and individuals may find it difficult to delimit the impact of these anxieties on their everyday experience. Thus for example, workers and managers in a nuclear power plant are

Stress in Health Professionals. Edited by Jenny Firth-Cozens and Roy L. Payne
© 1999 John Wiley & Sons Ltd

aware that they are working in a potentially dangerous environment, and nurses, physicians and administrators cannot ignore the fact that every day they are the witness to, or the makers of, life and death decisions. In these settings people are exposed to the anxiety that other people stimulate or to situations beyond their control, which implicate them in risky or dangerous activity or portend untoward results.

When anxiety takes on this social character, organisations may develop social defences which protect people psychologically. Isabel Menzies-Lyth (1988) first developed this concept when studying nurses in a hospital ward. She asked, for example, why nurses often wake up patients to give them sleeping pills. She suggested that the mindlessness of such a routine helped nurses avoid feeling too connected to their patients. If a patient's condition worsened, or she or he died, nurses would be less burdened by feelings of grief. Thus the routine, while on the surface appearing irrational, has the latent function of helping nurses to manage their anxiety. Most importantly, people who enact a social defence cannot consciously articulate its latent purpose. If they could, the defence would lose its power to allay fear. This is the sense in which a social defence reflects the operation of unconscious processes in organisations. The organisation does not have an unconscious, but people do. They create social defences which become institutionalised in organisational practice. These practices, these defences, are the group representation of individuals' anxieties, and we will be using this model of thinking about organisations in our case study.

WHAT IS STRESS?

Stress, as a measure of organisational functioning, is like the body's temperature—it is an epiphenomenon, the result of many social processes that culminate in how pressured or stressed people feel at work. For example, members of an entrepreneurial team working in the proverbial "garage" 70 to 80 hours a week, facing a most uncertain future, may experience little stress. Instead they will experience excitement, passion and hope. By contrast, people working as clerks in an office may sit in comfortable chairs, have good benefits and good supervisors but may experience significant stress. Stress is linked to the narratives people design for themselves as explanations for their experience. If I am part of a start-up team then I belong to an elite group of still unrecognised champions whose future is unbounded. If I am a dissatisfied clerk, I am in a job that gets me nowhere and appears to contribute little to the quality of the service my company offers its customers. Thus we cannot make sense of stress unless we make sense of how people make sense.

In addition, people may not, and often do not, have conscious know-ledge of their own narratives. It is a feature of any culture that its members are unaware of the assumptions unique to it. These assumptions set the ground or the context for awareness and are therefore not easily available for scrutiny. It takes mental work for a person to be aware of how he or she is aware.

We apply this perspective on stress to the following case study. We do this by examining a retreat we conducted with a nursing vice president and her five direct reports. The team faced an inordinate amount of work and was palpably stressed. The nursing VP wanted a retreat to help her reconnect to her direct reports and help them rebuild their relationships to one another. We argue that their stress was not simply due to over-work, but rather to the protective role they played within the hospital system. In particular, we hypothesise that the nursing directors were protecting the hospital's executive team from what we call the team's own "strategic ambivalence."

NURSING AT METRO HOSPITAL

Consider the following case: We were asked to consult to a team consist-ing of the nursing vice president of a hospital, to be called Metro, and her five direct reports. Metro faced the familiar problems confronting hospi-tals throughout the United States. There were too many hospital beds in the region, hospitals competed for patients and managed care companies were purchasing services from hospitals at low prices. When we were first contacted by the vice president for nursing, let us call her Joan, Metro senior executives had recently laid off many nurses and the resulting discontent led the remaining nurses to vote to form a union to represent them. In this same period, prior to Joan's joining Metro, Paula, a senior nurse, was the acting VP but because of family concerns was not willing to step into the full-time role.

When Joan took her job, the hospital was having difficulty recruiting and retaining nurses. This was due in part, as Joan discovered, to ac-tivities of an unqualified nurse recruiter but there was no doubt that the layoffs and subsequent unionisation gave Metro a bad reputation as an employer. Interestingly, after the union was voted in, several experienced nurses quit because they thought nurse professionals should not belong to a union. In addition, just at the moment that we began our interviews, Joan fired Carol, the head of a newly instituted unit of systems improve-ment, while Paula, the acting VP, left to live in another city. The directors did not complain openly about Carol's firing—we explore its rationale and meaning later in this chapter.

Finally, the Metro staff was preparing for a visit from the Joint Commission for Accreditation of Healthcare (JCAH), the national accrediting organisation that sets the standards for hospital care. In every hospital we have encountered, preparing for a JCAH visit is invariably time consuming and stressful. Hospital staff must review all their practices, identify deficiencies and correct them before the accrediting team arrives. Moreover, each hospital receives a numerical grade (up to 100) which is made public. The directors all felt that Metro was unprepared for the visit and they, as nursing directors, were now making up for lost time.

When Joan first asked us to consult she told us how stressed the nursing directors, as a team, appeared to be. The events of the last year were certainly tumultuous, she and her directors needed a "timeout", a place to think together and assess how they were doing. While at first Joan hoped to invite directors from other divisions of the hospital to the retreat, she decided, wisely we believe, to limit it to the people who reported directly to her. Feeling beleaguered already, she judged that her team would feel stressed to have "outsiders" attend the meeting, they needed a place where they could simply reconnect to each other.

To prepare for the one-day retreat we interviewed Joan's direct reports and several directors of other divisions, e.g. facilities and the cafeteria. We wrote a working note highlighting the themes we garnered from our interviews and circulated it to Joan and her staff before the retreat. During the retreat we took up facilitative roles, prodding, pushing and interpreting where we thought we could be helpful. The retreat was rich and nuanced, and revealed how people made sense of their experience and how this sensemaking helped or did not help them cope with the requirements of their work. Themes emerged—and we will explore each one in turn.

OVERFUNCTIONING

There is little doubt that the nurses and the nursing directors were very pressed for time. We want to highlight how nurses interpreted the scope of their obligations to Metro. Joan opened the retreat with the following thoughts:

> Today is a chance for us to step away and reflect. We are a magnet group. We draw the work to ourselves because we produce and deliver. Each of us has a major, major role. We are always at the table. . . . The JCAH is an overlay. Let's get ahead of the curve for the next time [they visit]. We have competition. We're vulnerable. Anything under the high 90s [the JCAH score] will affect our market share. How well we do is key to our viability.

The goal of today is to strengthen our workgroup, come away with how to prioritise. I worry about us being a team. I want us to be supportive of each other. I fear silos.

Joan is highlighting the sources of stress her team faces. Competition makes them vulnerable, and though they are unprepared for the JCAH visit, the stress that competition creates will not go away with better preparation. In addition, she suggests that because the team is so productive it literally draws work towards itself.

Later in the retreat Joan clarifies the role that nursing plays in reinforcing its magnet-like pull on work. Talking about the struggle she faces in setting priorities for her and the team, she notes:

I guess you can say I see everything as related to everything else. It's hard to prioritise when you see things that way. Everything is a priority and I fear leaving us absent from the table. *Also I have no confidence yet in giving some of our work to others: Will they do it right?*

In other words nursing suffers from overwork in part because the nursing staff, within the hospital and indeed the nursing profession within the culture of health care, still has second-rate status. Unless it actively takes up work or volunteers for extra work, it may be ignored when critical decisions are made. Moreover, since nurses effectively run the hospital day by day, they can ill afford to be absent from the table. The nurse directors suffer from overwork partly because they are struggling to secure their right to influence decisions.

Moreover, consider Joan's next statement:

It seems there are things we do for the department and other things that we do for the institution . . . [Certain political celebrities] are coming and we are getting involved there. We are magnets, martyrs, change agents.

Joan has now added the term "martyrs" to the word "magnet" she used to open the retreat. Martyrs willingly take up their role, even if it causes them pain. This suggests that in accepting their burdens the nurses are not simply victims but they actively create the overwork that then burdens them. The term "overfunctioning" is helpful here. First used in describing the role a family member might take up in a family, it points to a common organisational phenomenon as well. Certain people or groups take up the work that others should be performing. In this way they protect the under-performing person or group. The question becomes who or what is nursing protecting?

STRATEGIC AMBIVALENCE

Consider the following: the group was discussing the difficulties they were having in developing "clinical pathways", protocols for describing how a patient with a particular condition should be treated. Hospitals are introducing clinical pathways as a way of rationalising how care should be done. Invariably these pathways, when implemented, affect how physicians, as well as nurses, work. Betty, the director of the general medical and surgical unit, asks: "Why is it taking so long to develop clinical pathways? Some pathways are taking two years." Joan answers:

> There's a fear of revenue loss from more efficient pathways. We will be developing some, but it's not clear which. We will have one for asthma—perhaps the critically ill or out-patient. Out-patient means we will need community programmes, referrals from the schools. The institution will have to make itself more attractive to the asthma market. Consulting company X is coming in to build financial scenarios. If we drove asthma into out-patient what would it mean for revenues?

This answer, said without fanfare, points to an important dilemma, indeed we can call it a "strategic ambivalence". The Metro executive team was assuming, along with the leaders of many other hospitals, that, increasingly, insurers would pay hospitals a fixed fee per head to care for the health of people enrolled in the insurance plan. Hospitals would get the same amount of money per person whether that person used the hospital's in-patient services or not. Under these conditions, hospitals have every incentive to cut costs and decrease length of stay, because the number of hospital days is not connected to total revenue in any way. The executive team created a vision of the hospital as an integrated health system where services would be delivered, cost was lowest and quality highest.

Despite these assumptions, Metro and many other hospitals in the region had far fewer patients enrolled in these "capitation" plans than once expected. Hospitals, preparing hurriedly to create systems of care appropriate for capitation systems of payment, did not track people's resistance to these plans. As this essay is being written for example, there is a significant backlash against health maintenance organisations in the USA as people resist losing the right to choose which specialists they consult for their health problems and which hospitals they enter for treatment. Despite the executives' image of the hospital as an integrated health care delivery system designed for the capitation system, the truth was that the hospital faced a real risk in reducing costs. Paid on a per-diem basis, or for procedures performed, the hospital could make money by prolonging people's hospital stay or by seeing them on an in-patient rather than an out-patient basis.

When we interviewed Joan prior to the retreat she noted that she has experienced "resistance" from physicians and administrators when her staff worked on clinical pathways, but she characterised this resistance as puzzling or peculiar. Similarly, after the retreat, when we talked with her about capitation, she thought that the revenues Metro obtained from capitation plans were much higher than they actually were. It is sensible to ask how Joan, a woman of great talent and ability, could be so confused. After all, in responding to Betty she is quite clear: "There is a fear of revenue loss from more efficient pathways". In other words, if we do our job, Metro could lose money.

We think it useful to interpret Joan's confusion as a sign that the executive team had not yet confronted its own confusion. Instead, they "acted it out" by reinforcing the nursing work to develop clinical pathways and by permitting physicians and administrators to resist this work. We do not believe this is a trivial matter since it went to the heart of the executives' planning for Metro's future: how could it, how would it, make money?

Let us propose the following hypothesis: *The nursing staff was protecting the executive team and others from the confusion they were facing but were thus far denying.* Physicians and others who worried about the loss of revenue could blame nursing rather than the confused administration. This suggests that the stress the nursing directors felt was not simply due to overwork in the simple quantitative sense, but to working in an environment of contradiction and ambivalence. In other words, when people feel very clear about the purpose of their work they can tolerate the burdens imposed by the great amount of work they have to accomplish. When the work they do appears to be at cross-purposes with other work they do, or the work others are doing, this same quantity of work is experienced as much more stressful.

We think that this strategic ambivalence created another source of stress. Why might the executive team deny its own confusion? At one level we can ascribe this to the executives' common tendency to "keep their options open" and not make decisions. However we think their ostensible confusion was linked to moral questions as well. The vision of an integrated health care system is so attractive to health professionals because it gives them permission to treat people where they can best be helped. Hospital stays are a burden no matter how well the hospital environment is managed. Hospitals are iatrogenic institutions that can hurt people as they help them. Patients are away from home, are liable to get infected and the longer they stay the more likely they are to be victims of an error. The integrated health care system promises to marry considerations of cost and revenue with the moral impulse to treat patients in ways that are best for them, not simply good for the hospital. This suggests that one reason Joan appeared uninformed, and the executive team apparently confused, is that the moral vision of an integrated health system was itself so appealing. Just as nurses protected the executive team, they were helping to protect everyone's moral impulses, including their own.

OVERPROTECTION

The theme of protection played a central role throughout the retreat. As we conducted our interviews for the retreat, we were struck by how much the directors respected and appreciated Joan. As we wrote in the note circulated prior to the retreat:

> We detect not a whiff of cynicism about Joan. Our interviews with her directors indicate enormous goodwill ten months into her tenure, well past the honeymoon stage. People like and respect that she knows what she wants and tells them what she expects of them. She talks straight and people believe she listens. People say she is supportive and cares about their development. "A generous spirit", one person called her. "A shining star", said another, and a "light at the end of the tunnel".

This respect, indeed love, for Joan has created difficulties. Since her staff is eager to please her, it protected her from any difficulties she faced in creating priorities. At the end of the day, each member of the retreat, including Joan, reflected on what she had learned. Joan said:

> I learned that there needs to be more clarity around priorities. Perhaps I should have narrowed our goals for this year.

Joan could have failed to create more focused priorities because her staff could not refuse her any request. As Audrey, the director of one of the three intensive care units, said to Joan:

> You make me want to please you. So everything feels like a priority, I keep raising my own bar. It's like getting a notice in the mail: "Your credit card limit has been increased." I assume I should be able to make it all happen.

Throughout the retreat the team clarified how Joan's ability to say "no" to her peers was directly linked to her staff's ability to say "no" to her.

Joan noted that the Chief Executive Officer had asked her to straighten out the home health care service but that she turned it down. She said, "I said no," and the group actually applauded. Shortly afterwards, one consultant asked the group:

> Should Joan be holding the boundaries tighter so that the hospital doesn't pull her people out? Should she be the sayer of "no"?

Joan responded:

> I know I am not managing the boundary enough, but we will be held accountable for failure.

And this exchange unfolded:

> CONSULTANT: Is nursing overfunctioning? If so, this is a broader organisational development problem for the hospital. How can we bring this forward as an issue for the hospital as a whole? It's not something that can be resolved here.
>
> JOAN: I worry, am I becoming too controlling? I kept the Performance Improvement Unit in the face of some people saying it should go elsewhere . . .
>
> BETTY: The VP for nursing used to not be respected. Joan is, but the danger is that they will ask for too much.
>
> JOAN: It's not expected and customary for me to challenge the Chief Financial Officer, to fight for budgetary needs and so on.
>
> KATE (head of two of the three Intensive Care Units): I think you're defining the role.
>
> AUDREY (head of the third ICU): If you can say no to home health care, it lets me know that we can say no to you.

This is a rich interchange. In response to the consultant's query about overfunctioning, Joan reveals the complexities she faces in taking up her role. She may fail to protect her subordinates because she wants to sweep too much within her sphere of control. If she does this in part because she is overfunctioning, she is taking up work out of anxiety or insecurity. Joan notes that traditionally the VP for nursing does not challenge the Chief Financial Officer, in other words does not ask for more resources commensurate with the work nursing is expected to shoulder. Betty believes, though, that Joan is getting to the point where she can fight for more resources. Then Audrey notes that because Joan could exercise power by saying no to the home health care task, she can say no to Joan when Joan herself fails to set priorities. The interchange reveals the dynamics of an "overprotection" circle. Faced with pressure for work, and anxious about the status of nursing, Joan may say "yes" to inappropriate requests for work. This leads her to ask for more work from her directors, and because they so appreciate her leadership, they say "yes" to her. As Lucy suggests, this circle can be broken when Joan exercises power enabling the directors to exercise power as well.

Overprotection also emerged as a way group members tended to treat each other at the retreat. They were in some respects too gentle with each other. Consider the following interchange.

> MARCIA (the new director of the systems improvement unit): *I have huge shoes to fill and I'm worried about that.*
> BETTY: *Don't worry about the shoes. People know and respect you.*
> MARCIA: *The staff is questioning what is going on.*
> CONSULTANT: *This is a tension that will show up throughout today. The impulse to calm each other down versus working at the edge makes us anxious. We can be sensitive to switching back and forth. But let's try to work some at the edge.*

Marcia expresses concern, Betty tries to calm her down, but Marcia does not want to be protected, she wants to he heard. She rephrases her worry—"The staff is questioning what is going on".

This same process happened a second time when Winnie, the head of the social work department, expressed some of her concerns. During the period of retrenchment the social work department lost many of its cases and case workers, to the point that Winnie felt that the remaining workers might feel redundant.

> WINNIE: *Social workers often have a martyr complex. I think, aah, there can be some relief. But then there's my anxiety: will the institution need us any more?*
> MARCIA: *Social work is so valuable. Stop worrying.*
> CONSULTANT: *Let's push for not calming each other down. Let's stay with the risk.*

Marcia calms Winnie and the consultant once again intervenes, advocating that team members support each other to take risks. Interestingly, it was Marcia who did not wish to be calmed down the first time, but the pull to protect is sufficiently strong in the team's culture that Marcia, out of awareness, treats Winnie in the very way she herself did not wish to be treated—too gently.

The very nature of the nursing profession is to nurture and protect. It is therefore sensible that the directors would get pulled in this direction. We suggest here, however, that the Metro executive staff had hitchhiked on this natural tendency, this valence for protection, to protect themselves from their own confusion and fears. The nursing directors, in turn, internalised this protecting role they brought into the culture of the group so that they protected one another even when particular members wanted truth telling and frankness rather than protection.

POWER

We suggested that when Joan exercised power by saying "no", it helped her directors exercise power by saying "no" to her. Saying "no" was the way the nursing directors could begin to exercise some control over their work, and reduce the chances that they would suffer the stresses associated with overfunctioning. However, as is evident from the history of the nursing profession, nurses have an ambivalent relationship to power. On the one hand, nurses historically built a quasi-military organisation—a uniformed service—with the charge nurse and head nurse taking up roles akin to corporals and sergeants. The discipline associated with this kind of organisation was necessary to some degree. Nurses were after all in charge of situations in which life and death were at stake. The quasi-military organisation assured quality care. In addition, this form of work organisation partly relieved nurses from the guilt they would inevitably feel when patients died. After all they were at risk of blaming themselves for their own helplessness in the face of death. The quasi-military organisation depersonalised their work a bit. This is why, as Isabel Menzies-Lyth pointed out in a classic article on the psychodynamics of nursing (1988), nurses practised in a way that defied their caring impulses, e.g. waking up patients to give them a sleeping pill because it was the ordained time to do so.

   On the other hand, nurses always played second fiddle to physicians, board members and top administrators. Physicians controlled patient flow and determined the basic course of treatment, and the sex segregation of the profession—most physicians were men and almost all nurses were women—meant that nurses faced the dilemmas women feel exercising power in a male-centred society. Clearly these forces are attenuating. More women are becoming physicians, nurses have achieved more recognition for their clinical competence and many have become top administrators. Finally, the quasi-military structure of the nursing organisation is weakening. The terms ward, charge nurse and head nurse are losing ground to such terms as nursing manager and patient care manager. At the same time that hospitals become organised along product lines, e.g. cardiac care, pulmonary disease, etc., nurses are linked less to their own chain of command and more to health care teams, composed of physicians and other health professionals.

The past is not easily relinquished and we believe that the nursing directors at Metro still face difficulties in exercising power. Let us return to the case of Carol, the nurse who once headed up the systems improvement group and whom Joan fired.

This was a painful episode for Joan. Carol was, by all accounts, a brilliant woman with a vision of how clinical pathways, case management and systems for ensuring the continuity of care could revolutionise health care. However, the clarity of her vision was matched, not accidentally, by the aggression with which she pushed her ideas. Physicians and administrators began complaining to Joan about Carol, and when the volume of complaints became intolerable, Joan had to let Carol go.

During the retreat we brought up the question of what the directors might learn from Carol's experience. The directors did not want to consider this question. In some ways Carol's passion had infused the work of the nurses who filled the new case manager roles she had created, but this passion, while it animated the case managers, led others to feel that they were behaving as a new nursing elite. Carol unwittingly was creating dissension. After we raised the question for the third time Joan quite pointedly noted that Carol failed because she pursued her ideas "singularly". In other words, she lacked the political skills to build a consensus for her ideas.

We have no doubt that Joan was right but do not believe that was the whole story. It is a common experience for consultants to wrestle with the issue of why a client ignores a certain question the consultant asks. Is the consultant simply off base or is the client "resisting"? There is no formula we can use to answer this question. We suggest here that resistance did play a role. Carol, we could say, represented the hazard a nurse faces in exercising aggression. Joan, to be sure, could say "no", but she had the gift of saying "no" and pushing back with inordinate grace. In this sense she was the exception and this is why she was so admired. We suspect that the nurses could more readily identify with Carol, and her failure was a reminder that nurses, however committed or however visionary, could get burned if they exercise aggression.

We believe that we were inducted into the team's ambivalent feelings about the exercise of power. It affected how we took up our own roles. After we conducted the interviews we too felt overwhelmed by the amount of work the nursing directors had to accomplish. One of the directors, in fact, pleaded with us not to create more work for them as a result of the retreat. We decided that we could not give the entire retreat over to reflections and assessment, but had to carve out time in which the directors could accomplish work they had to do in any case, e.g. prepare for the JCAH visit. We explained our decisions to ourselves by assuring ourselves that we could observe the process of the directors working together and give them insight into their work-group culture without asking them to sacrifice valuable time.

In retrospect we believe this was a rationalisation. We felt gun-shy about demanding that they work in the spirit we think is most useful—to take time off to explore their identity, their assumptions and their working relationships. Yet as the retreat unfolded it became clear that the directors were more than ready to suspend their work-a-day work and use the retreat as a "retreat"—a place to withdraw from the work and think about how they work together and why. In other words, we did not exercise the aggression we needed to stand up for our own principles of consultation.

Finally, we think it is not an accident that Carol was in part extruded precisely around the issues that reflected the executive team's strategic ambivalence. She was pushing a vision of care most suitable for a funding environment shaped by capitation. It was not that she was simply being aggressive. Rather she was being aggressive on a set of initiatives the executive team and physicians were pursuing in a contradictory fashion.

STRESS ONCE AGAIN—AND THE TAVISTOCK APPROACH

Let us review our argument. We suggested that stress should not be thought of as a quantitative variable. Instead it is linked to how people make meaning of the situation, to the narratives they construct to explain their experience. In the case of Metro Hospital, we believe the nurses had developed a narrative they deployed unconsciously rather than consciously. Applying the Tavistock perspective, we look for system dynamics in the construction of this narrative. At the heart of the narrative was a story of the protector role the nurses had to play at the hospital.

While nurses have a valance for the protector role due to the kind of work they actually do, the nurses were swept into particular dynamics at Metro. The executive team was quite confused about the hospital's future. The funding environment had not unfolded as they had expected but they had yet to develop a strategy for the hospital that reflected this surprising turn of events. Instead the executive team asked nursing to pursue and represent contradictory actions, to develop new methods of care while at the same time protecting old ones.

In the Tavistock perspective this is systemic risk, risk that extends beyond the individual to the system. Risk stimulates anxiety, which in this case could not be managed by the individual. When anxiety takes on this social character, the organisation develops social defences that protect people psychologically. The Metro nurses were called upon to play a role in an unconscious narrative as the protectors of the hospital's flawed vision and the executive team's sense of efficacy.

This role shaped the nurses' own internal work culture. They protected each other from talking straight and they protected Joan, their leader, from the challenge she faced in setting priorities. Indeed, as we have seen, we too were drawn into this culture by protecting the nursing directors as a group from our own demands for work. Yet, as we have also seen, the group had great psychological resources. Afraid of losing time at the retreat, they nonetheless used it fully to explore their culture and to dig deeper into the important relationships between Joan and the group and between the group and the hospital.

REFERENCES

Czander, W.M. (1993). *The Psychodynamics of Work and Organizations: Theory and Application*. New York: Guilford Press.

De Board, R. (1978). *The Psychoanalysis of Organizations: A Psychoanalytic Approach to Behaviour in Groups and Organizations*. London: Tavistock Publications.

Hirschhorn, L. (1988). *The Workplace Within: Psychodynamics of Organizational Life*. Cambridge, MA: MIT Press.

Hirschhorn, L. (1992). *Managing in the New Team Environment: Skills, Tools and Methods*. Lexington, MA: Addison Wesley.

Hirshhorn, L. (1997). *Reworking Authority: Leading and Following in the Post-Modern Organization*. Cambridge, MA: MIT Press.

Menzies-Lyth, I. (1988). *Containing Anxiety in Institutions: Selected Essays*. London: Free Association Books.

Oblolzer, A. and Roberts, V.Z. (Eds) (1994). *The Unconscious at Work: Individual and Organisational Stress in the Human Services*. London: Routledge.

14

SHARING THE BURDEN: TEAMWORK IN HEALTH CARE SETTINGS

Angela J. Carter and Michael A. West

The current enthusiasm for teamworking in health care reflects a recognition that this way of working offers the promise of greater progress and support than can be achieved through individual endeavour and unstructured encounters with fellow workers. But, if people work in teams in health care settings, do they suffer less stress as a consequence? In this chapter we address this question by considering the research evidence, both within health care settings as well as in other sectors.

As workplaces and tasks become more complex and demanding, there is good evidence that working in teams enables people to more effectively meet the challenges of those tasks (Weldon and Weingart, 1993). Moreover, by working with others in team-based structures, people experience support as they attempt to cope with these demands (Sonnentag, 1996). However, the challenges of teamwork are also considerable and require specific skills and orientations among those attempting to work in this way. In this chapter we will explore the potential advantages of working in teams in health care settings; the obstacles both within the team and the wider organisational context; and we will examine practical ways of implementing team-based working within health care organisations.

Stress in Health Professionals. Edited by Jenny Firth-Cozens and Roy L. Payne
© 1999 John Wiley & Sons Ltd

Mohrman and colleagues (1995) define a team as:

> *a group of individuals who work together to produce products or deliver services for which they are mutually accountable. Team members share goals and are mutually held accountable for meeting them, they are interdependent in their accomplishment, and they affect the results through their interactions with one another. Because the team is held collectively accountable, the work of integrating with one another is included among the responsibilities of each member.*

In general, teams are used to achieve an aim or a goal that could not be accomplished easily, or possibly even at all, by an individual working alone. Midwives and health visitors have specialist skills which general practitioners do not and vice versa. Indeed, in most organisations, a mix of skills is required to provide complex services or produce sophisticated products. Mohrman *et al.* (1995) offer these reasons for implementing team-based working in organisations:

- Teams enable organisations to speedily develop and deliver products and services cost effectively, while retaining high quality.
- Teams enable organisations to learn (and retain learning) more effectively.
- Time is saved if activities, formally performed sequentially by individuals, can be performed concurrently by people working in teams.
- Innovation is promoted because of cross-fertilisation of ideas.
- Teams can integrate and link information in ways that an individual cannot.

The importance of teamworking in primary health care has been emphasised in numerous reports and policy documents on the National Health Service (NHS):

> *The best and most cost-effective outcomes for patients and clients are achieved when professionals work together, learn together, engage in clinical audit of outcomes together, and generate innovation to ensure progress in practice and service.* (NHSME, 1993)

Some limited research has suggested the positive effects of multidisciplinary teamworking in primary health care. In US studies, primary care teamworking has been reported to improve health delivery and staff motivation (Wood *et al.*, 1994) and to have led to better detection, treatment, follow-up and outcome in hypertension (Adorian *et al.*, 1990).

There is also evidence that teamworking can lead to a positive impact for the primary health care professionals themselves. In a study in Spain, Peiró *et al.* (1992) showed relationships between work team climate, role clarity, job satisfaction and leader behaviours. Effectiveness of teamwork was positively related to job satisfaction and the mental health of team members (correlations of 0.6 and 0.7 respectively). West and Wallace (1991), in a study of five innovative and three traditional UK primary health care teams, found that team innovativeness was positively related to team collaboration, commitment and tolerance of diversity of people and values within the team.

Teamwork and strain

A number of studies suggest that working in a team has a beneficial effect on team member mental health, including: a positive relationship between integrated working (workers who were more closely linked with fellow employees) and internal motivation (the extent to which employees gain self-esteem from successful job performance) in assembly and packaging workers (Moch, 1980); greater job satisfaction, involvement and commitment to the company's success in companies where teamwork and interdepartmental co-operation were high (Webb, 1989); improved job satisfaction and reduced sickness absence levels for nurses who were involved in team nursing (Boekhardt and Kanters, 1978); satisfaction associated with teamworking on an intensive care unit (Bilodeau, 1973); and lower reported strain among police officers working in teams (Greller *et al.*, 1992). There is some evidence, from America, that nurses working in self-managed units report improved well-being (in terms of increased job satisfaction and retention rates) when compared to units managed with more traditional hierarchical relationships (Weismann *et al.*, 1993). What impact does working in a team have on individual well-being? This is one of the research questions currently being investigated at the Institute of Work Psychology, University of Sheffield. This work looks at teams that provide primary and secondary health care and explores the well-being and effectiveness of these teams.

Teamwork and stress in primary health care

Primary health care is the first point of contact that people have with their health system. The composition of primary health care teams across the UK now varies from small general medical practices comprising one family doctor, receptionist and practice nurse, to large primary care networks, which include multiple family doctor partners, receptionist, managers, practice nurses and attached community nursing, health visiting, midwifery staff. Such networks may include nurse-practitioners, pharmacists, chiropodists, clinical psychologists and social workers.

What is the relationship between teamworking and stress in primary health care? As part of a project examining health care team effectiveness

(Borrill and West, 1998), we have studied a sample of 92 primary health care teams, via questionnaire surveys, videotaping of team meetings and focus group workshops. Questionnaire surveys have involved over 1,000 respondents. Using these data, we studied team processes and stress levels in 71 teams. Team sizes ranged from 5 to 66 members, with a mean team size of 21. There were highly significant differences between teams in terms of both team processes and strain (measured by scores on the General Health Questionnaire; GHQ-12, Goldberg, 1972). A score of 4 or more acts as an indicator of "minor psychological distress" (this is described as being a "case").

The overall case rate for GHQ scores was 21.8%, which is considerably lower than the average for health workers in secondary health care: Borrill et al. (1996) reported a mean GHQ score of 26.8% for a large group of NHS Trust employees. It is also somewhat lower than the GHQ caseness average for those working in teams in secondary care (mean GHQ score of 23%). The most highly stressed occupational groups were general practitioners, health visitors and practice managers. Those scoring lowest were community psychiatric nurses, midwives, professions allied to medicine, clerical workers and practice nurses. There was no relationship between team size and GHQ scores.

In order to determine whether team processes appeared to make a contribution to GHQ scores of the teams, we tested the significance of the effects of each of the team process measures (clarity of and commitment to team objectives; levels of participation, task orientation, task reflexivity and support for innovation). Each of these predictors was linearly related to GHQ at the team level, ranging from clarity of objectives, -0.31, $p<0.01$; through to task orientation, -0.45, $p<0.001$. In other words, the more positive the team processes the better the mental health of those working within teams.

Of course one explanation for these findings is that the results are due to "common method variance". That is, because we measured team processes and mental health using a similar method (self-report questionnaire responses) at the same time point, some of the relationship may be due to this common method of gathering the data. Alternatively, it could just be measuring an overall "feel good" effect—people feeling positive about life generally will be inclined to rate their own well-being positively and thus rate their teams very positively.

One way of addressing this issue is to consider the impact of interventions to promote teamworking within primary health care and then to determine whether the mental health of team imembers also improves. We have conducted such interventions with 10 primary health care teams. These involved working with teams over a six month period to help them define objectives using health needs analysis (i.e. defining the health needs of the local population, prioritising these and then defining team objectives relevant to these priorities). We also focused on improving levels of participation within teams (participation refers to interaction of information sharing, and with influence over decision making in teams). This was accomplished by encouraging those in positions of power (general practitioners, nursing managers) to devolve managerial responsibility down to members of the team. We also focused on improving team meetings. Task orientation was promoted by encouraging team members to examine critically the allocation of their team resources (including human resources) and to determine how best they could allocate these resources in order to meet prioritised health care needs. Team members engaged in a critical self-reflection debate, and appraisal, in order to determine how best their tasks could be performed collectively and objectives achieved. Finally, to facilitate support for innovation we invited team members to develop new and improved ways of working and to develop the necessary training and skill development required for them to meet the prioritised health needs of their local populations.

Figure 14.1 shows the before and after improvements in team processes following six-month interventions (which usually included six one-day workshops with each team), based on reports from 130 members of the 10 teams. Team processes can be seen to improve markedly. Figure 14.2 also shows the related improvements in mental health among team members following these interventions.

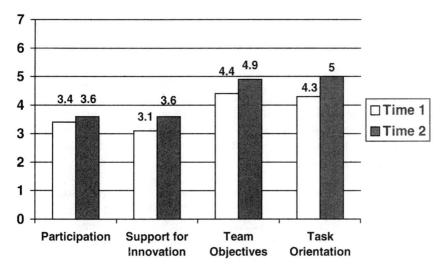

Figure 14.1: Improvement in team functioning following team interventions over a six-month period

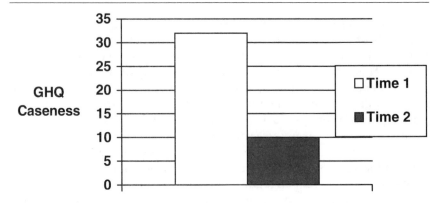

Figure 14.2:   Change in GHQ caseness following a six-month intervention

These results suggest that sustained interventions designed to encourage more effective teamworking lead to improvements both in team processes and team member mental health. While the improvements in team functioning are small, they are nevertheless consistent across teams and across all measures of team functioning. This suggests that, although the change is not large, it is consistent and reliable, reflecting real changes in team functioning, reported by members across the team.

TEAMWORK AND STRAIN IN SECONDARY HEALTH CARE

Secondary health care teams are work groups in NHS Trusts which provide health care to those referred for medical care, maternity care or health screening. Many of these teams are based in hospitals, while some teams have an interface with community care organisations (whole district NHS Trusts and community NHS Trusts). While there has been a developing research literature regarding primary health care teams (e.g. West and Wallace, 1991; Poulton and West, 1993, 1994) there is little research exploring health care team functioning across the various professional and support occupations found in hospital and community Trusts.

As part of a large-scale stress survey of health care organisations in England (Wall *et al.*, 1997; Borrill *et al.*, 1996), we identified 193 secondary health care teams (1,237 individuals). These teams came from 10 NHS Trusts. There were six types of teams: 86 nursing care; 51 multidisciplinary; 29 management; 10 medical; 6 quality improvement; and 11 support. Team sizes ranged from 2 to 44, with a mean team size of 11.

We examined the level of strain in these teams using the General Health Questionnaire (GHQ-12; Goldberg, 1972). The mean caseness of those members of the 193 secondary health care teams was 23%. This compares with scores of 27% for secondary workers generally and 17% for the general working population (Wall *et al.*, 1997). The strain levels were similar for front-line teams providing direct patient contact and for those providing support services. In addition to information regarding the strain levels of the team, significant relationships were seen between the measures of team functioning (clarity of objectives and levels of participation, task orientation and support for innovation) and well-being. These relationships are all negative, implying that good team functioning is associated with higher levels of psychological well-being (i.e. lower GHQ caseness). These results prompted a second study to explore whether team members enjoy better well-being than those who do not work in a team.

We asked 2,263 health care workers from four NHS Trusts (2 teaching, 1 District General Hospital, and 1 Community Trust) to complete measures of job satisfaction and well-being (the GHQ). In addition, a short questionnaire asked participants if they worked in a team and, if so, invited them to identify the characteristics of this team. The participants were asked:

- Do you work as part of a clearly defined team?
- Does your team have relatively clear objectives?
- Do you frequently work with other team members in order to achieve these team objectives?
- Are there different roles for team members within this team?
- Is your team recognised by others in the Trust as a clearly defined work team to perform a specific function?

On the basis of responses to these items participants were grouped into three categories: individuals who do not work in a team; individuals who work in a team that does not fit the five listed criteria (these were described as pseudo-teams); and individuals who work as part of a clearly defined team. Of the 2,263 health care workers, 12.5% did not work in a team; 30.6% worked in a pseudo-team; and 56.9% worked in a clearly defined team. Figures 14.3 and 14.4 illustrate the differences between these groups with respect to well-being and job satisfaction.

Those who work in a poorly defined team (pseudo-team), or do not work in a team, are significantly more likely to report higher levels of psychological distress and lower job satisfaction than those who work in a clearly defined team.

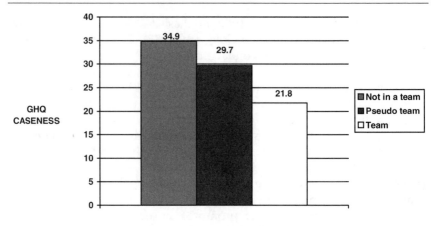

Figure 14.3:   Levels of strain

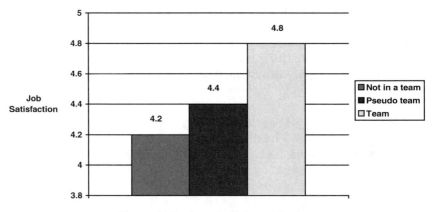

Figure 14.4:   Level of job satisfaction

OBSTACLES TO TEAMWORK IN HEALTH CARE

Our research clearly suggests the benefits of teamworking for the well-being of health care workers, and both researchers and policy makers have long urged teamwork on health care professionals as an effective way of promoting health care effectiveness.

Why then is the rhetoric of teamwork in health care not applied in practice? Below we consider historical obstacles created by the organisational context. Most health care professionals would recognise the need for interdependence and shared purpose, though studies have shown that there is little appreciation of the roles and responsibilities of other professionals (Poulton, 1995) and that primary health care professionals experience both role ambiguity and role conflict (Slater, 1996). Indeed, difficulties associated with co-ordinated teamworking were recognised in national reports (Department of Health and Social Security, 1986) which reviewed community nursing services in England and concluded that many primary health care teams exist in name only:

> *Separate lines of control, different payment systems leading to suspicion over motives, diverse objectives, professional barriers and perceived inequalities in status, all play a part in limiting the potential of multiprofessional, multi-agency teamwork . . . for those working under such circumstances efficient teamwork remains elusive.* (Audit Commission Report).

The piecemeal development of health care over its history has led to a number of structural, historical and attitudinal barriers standing in the way of efforts to promote teamwork in health care. More specifically, the problems include: separate lines of management; lack of an agreed model of leadership; lack of professional mutual role understanding and respect; dominance of physicians and the medical model; lack of understanding of organisational factors affecting teamwork; lack of pre-qualification teamworking training for professionals in primary health care; lack of clear team objectives and feedback on performance; failure of many teams to establish even the minimum of opportunities for team meetings and team reviews of strategies, processes and objectives; the unmet need to base practice and teamwork on strategic identification of health needs of local populations; and deep historical professional divisions, exacerbated by gender differentiation, which characterise the health care context (West and Slater, 1996, p. 29).

Such issues of professional division, status and gender differences are highly salient in health care teams. Further, different socialisation processes between doctors and nurses and separate basic and post-basic training for health care professionals are significant in shaping attitudes towards teamwork. Stokes (1994) suggests that attitudinal barriers to teamworking, which function at an unconscious level, are a product of these different backgrounds and training which shape values, attitudes and priorities. Medical training involves institutionalised and prolonged dependency of junior doctors on their seniors, from which the doctors eventually emerge to defend their new independence. This can degenerate into a counter-dependent state of mind, denying the mutual interdependency of teamwork and the actual dependency on the institutional setting of general medical practice.

Of critical importance to effective team functioning is organisational context. Scholars of teamworking across a variety of settings have come to the conclusion over recent years that the concern of social scientists with internal team processes to the neglect of the understanding of the organisational context within which teams work, is unhelpful. The organisational context plays a powerful role in shaping the effectiveness of teams (Mohrman *et al.*, 1995). Health care organisations, in order to encourage effective teamwork, have to provide:

- *Clear goals for teams* These goals should be related to the overall objectives of the organisation but should be negotiated with teams so that they are appropriate to local circumstances and reflect the team's knowledge of local needs.
- *Organisational reward for teams* Organisations tend to recognise and reward individual performance rather than recognising the performance of teams. This undermines the effectiveness of teamworking within the organisation.
- *Training for the job and training for teamwork* In health care organisations, understandably, there is almost exclusive concern with technical and professional training. However, to enable people to work effectively in teams requires that there is specific training for working in teams and the development of teamwork competencies (West and Allen, 1997).
- *The necessary process assistance to support the team in its work* In some teams, particularly those where members have a history of separate professional development and where status differentials are an obstacle, some process assistance may be necessary. In any team, there are times when conflicts or difficulties are impeding the group's work to such an extent that external assistance is required. Having such process assistance available within the organisation is important if teamwork is to be maintained, sustained and developed.
- *A supportive organisational climate* The organisational climate should be one which is supportive of people in teamworking. A concern with development, relationships, morale, commitment and inclusion and where there is a commitment to good communication, co-ordination and co-operation is required for effective teamworking within organisations. This is particularly so because teamworking functions best where there is a relatively flat hierarchy.
- *Supportive relations between teams in the organisation* Teamworking will be more effective in health care organisations where relationships between teams are mutually supportive—co-operative rather than competitive. Intergroup competition within health care organisations is likely to significantly undermine the organisation's effectiveness. Indeed, Mohrman *et al.* (1995) point out that one of the biggest causes of failure of team-based working is encouraging a climate of

intragroup development at the expense of intergroup co-operation. Consequently, teams begin to compete for resources and focus on their own effectiveness to the exclusion of the effectiveness of other teams within the organisation. This effectively undermines the effective functioning of the whole organisation. Therefore it is important that there are sufficient liaison and integrating devices between teams to ensure that they function effectively. This can include joint working parties, cross-team membership and representative teams with individuals from each team coming together on working groups to ensure effective co-operation and liaison.

The evidence that we have presented suggests that teamworking appears to buffer health professionals against the inevitable stresses associated with the content of their work. However, the organisational context of health care is a significant barrier to teamworking. Historical professional divisions, status hierarchies and an organisational context within which people are not encouraged to work in teams all impede collaborative working. The key to developing effective teamworking within health care settings is to ensure that organisations are restructured and processes are changed to encourage and support teamworking. This requires a vision from the top of health care organisations and a commitment from those throughout organisations to bring about these changes, to achieve co-operative, interdependent working and ultimately better health care for the whole community.

REFERENCES

Adorian, D., Silverberg, D.S., Tomer, D. and Wamasher, Z. (1990). Group discussions with the health care teams: a method of improving care of hypertension in general practice. *Journal of Human Hypertension*, **4**(3), 265–268.

Audit Commission (1992). *Homeward Bound: A New Course for Community Health* (p. 20). London: HMSO.

Bilodeau, C.B. (1973). The nurse and her reactions to critical care nursing. *Heart and Lung*, **2**(3), 358–363.

Boekhardt, M.G. and Kanters, H.W. (1978). Team nursing in a general hospital: theory, results and limitations. *Journal of Occupational Psychology*, **51**(4), 315–326.

Borrill, C.S., Wall, T.D., West, M.A., Hardy, G.E., Shapiro D.A., Carter, A.J., Golya, D.A. and Haynes C.E. (1996). *Mental Health of the Workforce in NHS Trusts*. Published by the Institute of Work Psychology, University of Sheffield.

Borrill, C.S. and West, M.A. (1998). *Strain in Primary Health Care*. Unpublished report. Institute of Work Psychology, University of Sheffield.

Department of Health and Social Security (1986). *Neighbourhood Nursing—A Focus for Care (The Cumberledge Report)*. London: HMSO.

Goldberg, D.P. (1972). *The Detection of Minor Psychiatric Illness by Questionnaire*. Oxford: Oxford University Press.

Greller, M.M., Parsons, C.K. and Mitchell, D.R.D. (1992). Additive effects and beyond: occupational stressors and social buffers in a police organisation. In J.C. Quick, L.R. Murphy, & J.J. Hurrell Jr (Eds) *Stress and Well-being at Work: Assessments and Interventions for Occupational Mental Health*. American Psychological Association.

Moch, M.K. (1980). Job involvement, internal motivation, and employees' integration into networks of work relationships. *Organisational Behaviour and Human Performance*, **25**, 15–31.

Mohrman, S.A., Cohen, S.G. and Mohrman, A.M. (1995). *Designing Team-Based Organizations*. San Francisco: Jossey-Bass.

NHSME (1993). *Nursing in Primary Health Care—New World, New Opportunities*. Leeds: National Health Service Management Executive.

Peiró, J.M., Gonzalez-Romá, V. and Ramos, J. (1992). The influence of work team climate on role, stress, tension, satisfaction and leadership perceptions. *European Review of Applied Psychology*, **42**(1) 49–56.

Poulton, B.C. (1995). *Effective Multi-disciplinary Teamwork in Primary Health Care*. Unpublished PhD thesis. Institute of Work Psychology, University of Sheffield.

Poulton, B.C. and West, M.A. (1993). Effective multi-disciplinary teamwork in primary health care. *Journal of Advanced Nursing*, **18**, 918–925.

Poulton, B.C. and West, M.A. (1994). Primary health care team effectiveness: developing a constituency approach. *Health and Social Care*, **2**, 77–84.

Slater, J.A. (1996). *Occupational Stress in Primary Health Care*. PhD thesis. School of Nursing, University of Wales College of Medicine.

Sonnentag, S. (1996). Work group factors and individual well-being. In M.A. West (Ed.) *Handbook of Work Group Psychology* (pp. 345–367). Chichester: Wiley.

Stokes, J. (1994). The unconscious at work in groups and teams. In A. Obholzer and V.Z. Roberts (Eds) *The Unconscious at Work: Individual and Organizational Stress in the Human Services*. London: Routledge.

Webb, S. (Ed.) (1989). *Blueprint for Success: A Report on Involving Employees in Britain*. London: The Industrial Society.

Wall T.D., Bolden, R.I., Borrill, C.S., Carter, A.J., Golya, D.A., Hardy, G.E., Haynes, C.E., Rick, J.E., Shapiro, D.A. and West M.A. (1997). Minor psychiatric disorder in NHS Trust staff: occupational and gender differences. *British Journal of Psychiatry*, **171**, 519–523.

Weismann, C.S., Gordon, D.L., Cassard, S.D., Bergner, M. and Wong, R. (1993). The effects of unit self-management on hospital nurses' work process, work satisfaction, and retention. *Medical Care*, **31**(5), 381–393.

Weldon, E. and Weingart, L.R., (1993). Group goals and group performance. *British Journal of Social Psychology*, **32**, 307–334.

West, M.A. and Allen, N. (1997). Selection for teamwork. In N.R. Anderson and P. Herriot (Eds) *International Handbook of Selection and Assessment* (pp. 493–506) Chichester: Wiley.

West, M.A. and Slater, J. (1996). *The Effectiveness of Teamworking in Primary Health Care*. Oxford Health Education Authority.

West, M.A. and Wallace, M. (1991). Innovation in health care teams. *European Journal of Social Psychology*, **21**, 303–315.

Wood, N., Farrow, S. and Elliott, B. (1994). A review of primary health care organization. *Journal of Clinical Nursing*, **3**(4), 243–250.

15

GETTING THINGS RIGHT FOR THE DOCTOR IN TRAINING

Fiona Moss and Elisabeth Paice

INTRODUCTION

Doctors are at particular risk from experiencing work-related stress and depression, as other chapters in this book have made clear. These findings are not confined to doctors working in the UK and are not new (Firth-Cozens, 1987; McCue, 1985; Butterfield, 1988). There is some evidence from studies in the UK (Firth-Cozens, 1987) and the USA (Girard *et al.*, 1991) that doctors are most vulnerable to work-related stress in their first year of work—the pre-registration year in the UK or intern year in the USA—and that stress levels may decline over time and with seniority (Grainger *et al.*, 1996) Nevertheless studies have shown that stress, stress-related problems and depression persist at a higher level than in the general population throughout the medical career, both in hospital doctors and in general practitioners (Caplan, 1994; Firth-Cozens, 1997; Sutherland and Cooper, 1993).

Some of the work of doctors is invariably stressful and even the duty of responsibility that doctors have to their patients may in itself be a stressor. But undue stress, even in the short term, has a detrimental effect on an individual's performance at work and in the context of health care it may impinge on the delivery of good-quality care (Firth-Cozens and Morrison, 1989; McKee and Black, 1992). Reducing work-related stress or

Stress in Health Professionals. Edited by Jenny Firth-Cozens and Roy L. Payne
© 1999 John Wiley & Sons Ltd

minimising its effects is not only important for the health and well-being of doctors but also may also help to improve the quality of care received by their patients. In this chapter, we review some of the causes of stress on doctors in training—looking particularly at pre-registration house officers—and consider some of ways that stress can be reduced or counter-balanced by interventions that mitigate or neutralise the effects of stressors.

STARTING OUT RIGHT: PREPARATION FOR WORKING AS A DOCTOR

In the UK most medical students enter medical schools directly from school. Some will have had a gap year but few are graduates and few will have had experience of full-time employment before starting their studies. Starting your first job is a "life event", but for newly qualified doctors that first job also marks a crucial rite of passage—from being a student to being a doctor and entry into a profession. Thus, in addition to specific job-related stressors, the actual experience of starting full-time work may itself be a source of stress. For medical students starting work involves an enormous change in lifestyle and in outlook. They move from the largely self-focused life of an undergraduate to jobs that, by their nature, demand a high degree of responsibility for others; that are highly rostered and arduous; and that depend on the ability to work closely with and communicate with others. And there is little choice about when the newly graduated doctor starts his or her first post—in Britain all pre-registration posts start in August or February—or the types of jobs they must undertake at this stage.

Many newly qualified doctors feel that they are ill-prepared for the work of being a pre-registration house officer and experience a mismatch between the medical school curriculum and the skills and competencies they find they need as pre-registration house officers. The need for con-gruency between the medical school curricula and the skills and compe-tencies needed for work as a pre-registration house officer is acknowledged in the introduction to the General Medical Council's re-commendations for undergraduate medical teaching, *Tomorrow's Doctors*: "We must ensure . . . that the newly qualified doctor is well prepared for the responsibilities for the pre-registration house officer year." But simply including a topic in a course may not lessen its potency as a stressor. For example, although all medical schools now include teaching on death and dying and breaking bad news in their curricula, in a qualitative investiga-tion of the stress and coping in a group of pre-registration doctors the most frequently cited group of stressful events related to the care of people who were dying or concerned ethical issues (Firth-Cozens and Morrison, 1989).

In the principal recommendations of *Tomorrow's Doctors* it is stated that: "The *essential skills* required by the graduate at the beginning of the pre-registration year must be acquired under supervision, and proficiency in these skills must be rigorously assessed" (General Medical Council, 1992). Understanding what these "essential" skills are is crucial if the new curricula of the medical schools are to provide coherence between undergraduate experience and the needs of the newly qualified doctor. While clinical and technical skills are obviously essential, it is clear to those who work in hospitals—nurses and hospital managers as well as pre-registration house officers and consultants—that other skills are also important; for example, the ability to communicate well with staff and patients; organisational skills including teamworking; and personal skills such as time management and ability to prioritise (Moss and Miller, 1998). Graduates who understand these other non-medical technical skills may be better able to integrate into the world of hospital work and perhaps be less vulnerable to the effects of stress than those who have only acquired clinical skills. The timing of programmes that introduce these skills is crucial. The anxieties of medical students are different from those of qualified doctors and probably relate more to perceived anxieties arising from current problems and situations (Moss and McManus, 1992). The skills and topics that might better prepare the student/graduate for the world of work that are clearly related to the context of the work and world of pre-registration house officers should be introduced at a time when their relevance is apparent: "just-in-time training". Those successfully introduced within the undergraduate course must continue to be the focus of learning within the pre-registration year.

A possible contributing factor to the high levels of stress experienced by doctors is that those who enter medicine are inherently more vulnerable to work stressors than others. There is some evidence that depression in some individual doctors predates career choice and that, for some individuals, these decisions may be related to individual characteristics such as high self-criticism or particular relationships with their parents (Firth-Cozens, 1997). Thus, given the current selection processes, there is a particularly strong case for ensuring that medical students are prepared adequately for the transition from the world and work of the undergraduate and that adequate induction is provided for doctors starting new jobs.

STARTING OUT RIGHT: INDUCTION

The beginning of a post provides an opportunity to help newly appointed doctors adjust to the work setting and to introduce them to sources of support within the team and the hospital. For the newly qualified doctor, who may be starting work for the first time, there are some important issues—e.g. where to get help—that should be made explicit at this time, and that may help to reduce vulnerability to stress and stressors. Induction programmes for new employees are standard practice in many organisations. Their aim is to help new employees to learn about the place of work and thus to settle down and work effectively in the new environment (Advisory Conciliation and Arbitration Service, 1987).

Induction programmes for pre-registration house officers were introduced in a few hospitals in the late 1980s. To be effective and useful to the newly appointed doctor they need to be planned carefully and the people with whom the new doctors will be working should be available to welcome them to their new work. An evaluation of the 1990 induction course at Lewisham Hospital, London, found that the only talk to make any impact was one by a departing house officer titled, "What is it like to be a house officer and how will I cope without making some dreadful mistake?" Realising that the course consisted of a series of talks given over four hours and that it met the needs of the hospital rather than the pre-registration house officers, the induction programme was redesigned. The new course is based on small groups led by outgoing pre-registration house officers with essential information provided in a handbook rather than transmitted in talks. The new induction also includes an introduction to the department or team, and an opportunity to meet the consultant with whom they will be working (Gale *et al.*, 1992; Jackson, 1998). Getting induction right so that it meets the needs of the new doctors should reduce anxiety at the start of a post and may mitigate early the effects of potential stressors.

The importance of induction is now recognised and since 1994 all pre-registration house officers have been required to start their August post a day before the previous cohort leave to enable all hospitals to meet a requirement to use that day for induction (NHS Management Executive, 1994). There is a growing appreciation of the need to arrange appropriate induction to every post and at every grade, especially if the post is the first the trainee will have undertaken in that specialty.

Whatever the preparation, starting a first post as a doctor is likely to be stressful:

> *Faces were familiar, I knew the daily routine and most importantly, I had a clear idea of what to expect and what was expected of me. I still woke up on the first day of work worrying about being first on the scene of a cardiac arrest or prescribing a lethal dose of a drug, but by lunch time I realised that by and large the day to day running of the ward continued despite me.* (Richardson, 1998).

It is important that those working with and supervising newly appointed doctors are aware of their needs, provide support, and help them to understand the workings of what is for them a new environment.

CONDITIONS OF WORK

Hours

The long hours worked by doctors, especially in first posts after graduating are often blamed for the stress and distress of being a "junior" doctor. However, in a cohort study of stress in pre-registration house officers, although *perceived overwork* was the most stressful aspect of pre-registration house officers' work, no relationship was found between levels of stress or depression and number of hours worked (Firth-Cozens, 1987). Long hours have been shown to be associated with a direct affect on current health in terms of somatic symptoms and social dysfunction, but may have a less damaging effect on well-being and perhaps fewer long-term sequelae than the type of demands made on doctors during those hours.

In the UK the hours doctors in training are obliged to work have been the focus of an important national programme: the "New Deal" (Department of Health, 1991). This is an initiative that has met with some success in that few doctors are now contracted to work for more than 72 hours a week, whereas before 1991 it was common to be expected to work for more than 83 hours a week. This intervention had a number of consequences. The amount of work did not diminish, so there was a tendency under the new system for the intensity of work to rise. To reduce the intensity, more doctors, especially senior house officers (SHOs), were employed, some traditionally medical tasks were taken on by nurses, phlebotomists and ward clerks, and patterns of work changed. An interview survey of SHOs in North Thames, before and after the introduction of the New Deal, revealed that while the intensity of work had increased, the combination of reduced total working hours and reduced inappropriate duties had removed the sense of being overwhelmed (Paice *et al.*, 1997).

Sleep deprivation

Sleep deprivation is a potent stressor. There is much evidence that links sleep deprivation with deterioration in mood and also with performance (Deary and Tait, 1987; Lingenfelser *et al.*, 1994). Sleep loss and sustained work have direct effects on performance but there are individual differences and their effects on performance may be mediated by mood (Firth-Cozens, 1993). For many decades doctors in training grades have had to work and make decisions about patients while suffering from lack of sleep (Masterton, 1965; Friedman et al., 1971). Levels of fatigue higher than those found in the general population have been found in health care workers (Hardy et al., 1997)—especially among doctors and other clinical professionals. General fatigue seems to be dependent on levels of psychological distress and high experienced work demands.

The "New Deal", in addition to setting out guidelines on the total number of hours that doctors should work, also established the minimum hours of uninterrupted sleep, and the minimum period an individual should be able to take off within a working schedule. One approach to meeting these targets has been to introduce work patterns based on shift systems. Shift working is appropriate in areas of care where the intensity and the type of work are similar throughout a 24-hour period and where patient stays are short—for example, intensive care, special care baby units, and accident and emergency departments. But shift working may not be appropriate in specialties whose work is mostly done in the daytime where the doctors also provide medical cover at night and are part of the rota for emergency admissions. Partial shifts, in which a basic daytime working pattern is maintained but where individuals take turns working late shifts or nights, is one approach to meeting targets on hours, sleep and off-duty periods. However, this approach to working has not proved universally popular and may limit continuity of care and team-working (Baldwin et al., 1997), both of which may be important mitigators of stress.

Minimising the sleep deprivation experienced by doctors in training is likely to benefit patient care as well as improve the well-being of the doctors. A small study in the USA looked at the effects of changing interns' and residents' work schedules so that sleep deprivation was reduced. Not only did this change in work pattern increase doctors' sleep but some aspects of patient care improved—fewer medication errors, shorter duration of stay, and fewer requests for laboratory tests (Gottlieb et al., 1991). While the precise schedules described may not be transferable, this small study illustrates the potential effects on patient care of minimising sleep deprivation.

Permitting sleep deprivation, or not allowing periods of rest and opportunity to catch up on sleep, suggests a fundamental institutional lack of concern for the well-being of individuals working within the health care system, with important consequences for patients. That is not to say that no one cares; they clearly do, but there are seen to be too many obstacles to improving the working life and conditions of a vulnerable group. The problem is clearly more than one of "hours" and the solutions are likely to require considerable organisational change. In one example, where the work and hours of senior house officers were considered in the context of the work of the whole unit, hours were reduced by recognising areas of duplication of work; looking at the needs of some groups of patients and making changes to the organisation and pattern of work of all doctors and nurses. One of the changes was the establishment of a daily open access clinic for referrals from general practice. The changes—which were felt most by the nurses—not only helped the doctors but also resulted in a 91% reduction in out-of-hours procedures (Read and Draycott, 1998).

Tasks

Tasks perceived as menial or repetitive are particularly associated with stress. Other specific work-related factors that contribute to young doctors' feelings of being overwhelmed include the number of emergency admissions and the number of deaths . Moreover, some young doctors may not be fully competent to undertake some expected tasks (Teahon and Bateman, 1993).

Inappropriate duties have been reduced. Most hospitals now have phlebotomists to take blood and the introduction of hospital information systems has increased easy access to results of clinical tests. Some tasks previously undertaken by doctors are now more usually done by nurses (Koay and Marks, 1996). But there may at times be confusion between nursing roles and the roles of newly qualified doctors (Chant, 1998) and there is always the possibility that removing one source of stress may introduce another.

Reducing the number of menial tasks is only part of the process. Newly qualified doctors should not be required to attempt tasks for which they have not been trained and should be trained to seek help when faced with situations they have not dealt with before. This is perhaps as much a matter of attitudinal change about roles among young doctors as it is of providing better support. Understanding task and role clarity has been found to be associated with greater job satisfaction and reduced stress among senior house officers in accident and emergency departments (Heyworth *et al.*, 1993). These are issues that could be included in an induction.

EXPERIENCE AND CLINICAL SUPERVISION

While the New Deal has been welcomed for reducing the stress associated with excessive hours of work and sleep deprivation, anxieties have been expressed by young doctors and their supervisors that they may not be gaining adequate experience. In a questionnaire survey of trainees of all grades and specialties (2,947 responses, response rate 71%; (Paice and Craig, 1997) the most frequent response to the question "What would most improve your post?" was "More hands-on experience". This was true of both pre-registration and senior house officers, but most particularly in the surgical specialties. High ratings for hands-on experience acquired in the post were not associated with the hours or intensity of work, or the amount of rest during a night on call. High ratings were, however, associated with high ratings for consultant supervision, and were associated with high levels of satisfaction with the post (Paice, 1998). Young doctors enjoy gaining hands-on experience in their profession, but this happens most effectively under appropriate supervision, within an educational framework, and when they are not too tired to learn.

Feeling forced to cope beyond experience or competence

Young doctors do not enjoy being "thrown in at the deep end", and are deeply conscious of the potential consequences of the serious mistakes they may make through ignorance or inexperience (Baldwin *et al.*, 1998). In a questionnaire survey done in 1996 in North Thames, doctors in training were asked how often they felt forced to cope, with problems beyond their competence or experience. There was an inverse relationship between feeling forced to cope, and satisfaction with the post, whatever the grade or specialty. The more junior the trainees, the more often they felt exposed. Over 50% of pre-registration house officers felt forced to cope once or twice a week or more often, compared with 30% of senior house officers and less than 20% of higher specialist trainees. But a good induction to the post, and good consultant supervision, were associated with fewer junior doctors feeling forced to cope with such problems (Figures 15.1–15.3).

EDUCATIONAL SUPERVISION

There is much evidence to link lack of feedback about progress, and poor educational supervision with high levels of stress (Firth-Cozens, 1987). In a survey that we have carried out in North Thames of over 1,000 pre-registration house officers, the level of supervision by middle grade doctors correlated with pre-registration house officers' overall satisfaction with their posts. Moreover, a major source of stress cited by pre-registration doctors is their relationship with senior staff (Richardson, 1998) . Analysis of the use of a logbook by pre-registration house officers

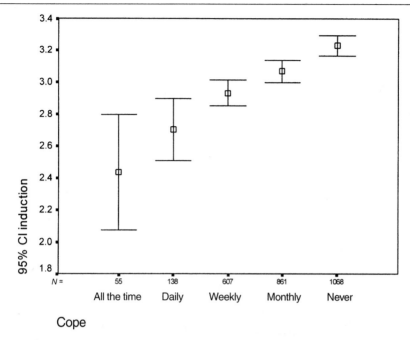

Figure 15.1: Responses to the question: "How often do you feel forced to cope with problems beyond your competence or experience?" against mean rating of induction to the post (with 95% confidence intervals) where 1 = very poor and 5 = excellent ($n = 2,729$)

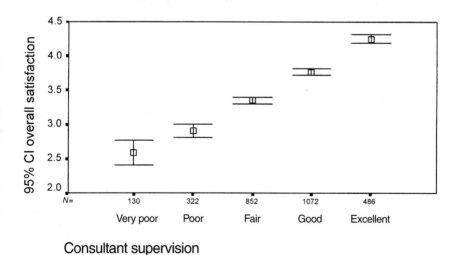

Figure 15.2: Relationship between consultant supervision and overall satisfaction (where 1 = very poor and 5 = excellent)

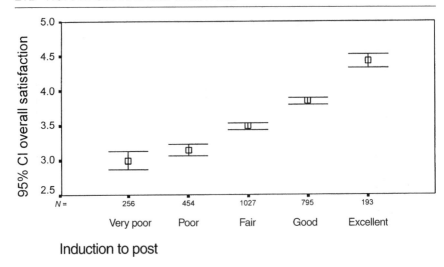

Figure 15.3:   Relationship between assessment of induction and overall satisfaction with post (where 1 = very poor and 5 = excellent)

demonstrated that trainees who had the opportunity to discuss the log book with their consultants were more satisfied with their jobs than others (Paice *et al.*, 1997). Until recently most junior doctors did not receive any feedback on progress (Garrud, 1990; Doherty *et al.*, 1992) but there has been a change in consultant behaviour, and our survey showed that regular appraisal sessions are becoming more common. Trainees who had not received feedback, or who had not found it useful, were more likely to feel forced to cope beyond their competence or experience, and more likely to plan to leave medicine (Paice, 1997). Putting these findings together identifies the consultant trainer as a potential source of support or stress. Helping consultants to become proactive and supportive trainers is, therefore, an intervention likely to improve job satisfaction and reduce stress in young doctors.

Our experience from interviewing many pre-registration house officers as part of the University of London's process of approving house officer posts, has demonstrated enormous variation in the support that consultants provide in terms of both supervision and feedback. Often pre-registration house officers have no idea about their attainment in these crucial first posts, and as many tend towards being self-critical (Firth-Cozens, 1997) the lack of feedback may be interpreted as suggesting lack of achievement. In her work on the experience of the pre-registration year, Dowling describes the fragmented support and supervision for pre-registration house officers provided by consultants (Dowling and Barret, 1991). But where consultant clinical supervisors take care to forge active and supportive relationships, the house officers are more satisfied with their posts (Figure 15.2) and, we would argue, less vulnerable to the effects of work-related stressors.

Many consultants have had no specific instruction in how to supervise, train and support doctors in training posts and bring to their supervisory and training roles their own experience of working in a training grade. The specific role of being a clinical supervisor or trainer is not distinguished separately from a consultant's clinical role. In general practice, however, only some general practitioners are trainers, and to become a trainer requires assessment of both the potential trainer and the practice in which he or she works.

Ideally, we would propose a system in which only those consultants with appropriate skills and experience who wanted to take on the extra role of being a clinical trainer would do so. But in the context of the organisation of hospital care, that is clearly not practicable. Introducing specific guidelines for consultant trainers and setting up programmes to enable consultants and senior specialist registrars to develop appropriate skills could be a very cost-effective intervention. It is disappointing that, so far, few of the curricula developed for specialist registrar training include preparation for the young trainee specialist's role as a future trainer.

SUPPORT FROM OTHER STAFF

The ward sister working mainly with one medical or surgical team is a figure whom many senior doctors cite as an important source of advice and support when they were newly qualified. But reduction in hospital beds, and pressure on remaining beds, means that most medical teams care for patients on several wards and do not have a clear working relationships with a particular group of nursing staff. The relationship between young doctors and nursing staff, all of whom are under considerable pressure, may have changed and the support available for both groups diminished. Active intervention is needed to rebuild multi-professional teams that will provide the necessary support for health care professionals—and thereby improve patient care. In a recent iniative in North Thames, some hospitals provide a nurse mentor, who has specific educational and supportive role for some pre-registration house officers. This is one approach to re-creating a multi-professional network of support that may help reduce the effect of stressors for pre-registration house officers.

ORGANISATION OF WORK

If clinical firms are to be reorganised to reduce work-related stressors, it is in our view crucial that any reorganisation is based on a coherent team structure. In those hospitals where clinical work is organised around clearly defined teams, individuals support each other. Senior house officers in accident and emergency medicine who view their work groups as cohesive appear more satisfied with their jobs and less stressed that those who experience less group cohesiveness (Heyworth *et al.*, 1993). Ideally, the clinical team should include nurses and other health care professionals. In our work with pre-registration house officers one of the factors most strongly associated with job satisfaction is whether or not they feel part of a team. The link between good teamwork and reduced stress is relatively newly recognised, but clearly is an important way forward.

Working out satisfactory ways of working that minimise stress and sleep deprivation for doctors will depend on understanding that, for many medical teams, there is a fusion of night and emergency work with routine daytime tasks such as out-patient clinics and endoscopy lists and that a large proportion of the work done by doctors at night could more safely and appropriately be left until the morning or done by non-medical staff (Dowling and Barret, 1991). Ten years ago a study on out-patient activity reported that it was not uncommon for doctors seeing patients in the out-patient clinic to have been on continuous duty for 24 hours (Kiff and Sykes, 1988). If duties are arranged so that doctors responsible for acute admissions do not have routine responsibilities at the same time, or the following day, doctors won't be put in the impossible, and stressful situation, of having simultaneous responsibility for two groups of patients. New approaches to the organisation of care appropriate for the needs of patients and for the well-being of health care professionals are needed (Paice and Ingham Clark, 1997). Sorting out schedules to provide an appropriate skill mix of staff at night is a matter of concern for all managers, senior nursing staff as well as doctors.

INDIVIDUAL COPING STRATEGIES

When considering interventions to reduce work-related stress it is important to realise that, despite the high stress levels experienced by doctors and the sometimes absurd demands of the work, many doctors in training find their work fulfilling and demonstrate the capacity to minimise the stress on themselves and to function well and healthily. Finding out what these doctors find fulfilling or enjoy most may help the search for ways to reduce stress in others. Moreover, it seems to us that there are some hospitals where doctors seem happier and less stressed than others. Understanding both these organisational differences may provide insight into factors that mitigate or reduce stress (Scott *et al.*, 1995)

The majority of coping strategies identified by pre-registration doctors as being used in association with a stressful event, can be classified either as simply "tackling the problem" or "asking for help" (Firth-Cozens and Morrison, 1989; Paice *et al.*, 1997). Stressed doctors are more likely than relatively unstressed colleagues to respond to stressful situations by "dismissing the event". (Firth-Cozens and Morrison, 1989; Paice *et al.*, 1997). If consultants and others who supervise the progress of house officers are aware of these different approaches to stress then they should be able to identify and help those more vulnerable to the effects of stresses.

Despite recognition of their stress, most doctors do not seek professional help but rely on family and friends for support. A few seek professional help and find it useful, but many more indicate that they would welcome informal counselling in the workplace (Scott *et al.*, 1995; King *et al.*, 1992). Some professional help is available—for example, the sick doctors help-line and the BMA telephone counselling service log many thousands of calls a year. In some regions postgraduate deans provide access to independent counsellors who will offer support on a one-to-one, confidential basis (Hale, 1998). However, doctors suffering from stress do not necessarily avail themselves of help. The reasons are probably that most stressed doctors do not see themselves as "sick" or in any way different from their colleagues. Furthermore, doctors rarely feel able to take time off work—even for physical problems (McKevitt *et al.*, 1997) Even encouraging doctors to express their feelings and to acknowledge difficulties would be an important step towards limiting the damaging effects of stresses.

CONCLUSIONS

Much of the work on the stress in health care workers has focused on the analysis of the problems experienced by doctors and the public debate has particularly concerned the legendary long working hours demanded of doctors in acute hospitals. But the causes of stress are much more complex than the sum of the hours worked. Strategies to reduce stress—if they are to be successful—will require a review of all aspects of clinical work and challenge old and set working practices as well as the work and roles of all health care professionals, not just the work of the doctors in training. More will be asked of consultants as trainers, and there must be increased support and supervision from all senior health care professionals. Making some of these changes will be difficult and will require an enormous change in attitude, a break with past experiences and expectations, and include radical reorganisation of working practices. But there is a prevailing mood for change.

REFERENCES

Advisory Conciliation and Arbitration Service (1987). *Induction Booklet*, No 7. ACAS.

Baldwin, P.P.J., Newton, R.W., Buckley, G., Roberts, M.A. and Dodds, M. (1997) Senior house officers in medicine: a postal survey of training and work experience. *British Medical Journal*, **314**, 740–3.

Baldwin, P.J., Dodd, M. and Wrate, R.M. (1998). Junior doctors making mistakes. *The Lancet*, **351**, 804.

Butterfield, P.S. (1988). The stress of residency. A review of the literature. *Archives of International Medicine*, **148**, 1428–1435.

Caplan, R.P. (1994). Stress, anxiety, and depression in hospital consultants, general practitioners and senior health service managers. *British Medical Journal*, **309**, 1261–1263.

Chant, A.D. (1998). A confusion of roles: manpower in the National Health Service. *Journal of the Royal Society of Medicine*, **91**, 63–65.

Deary, I.J. and Tait, R. (1987). Effects of sleep disruption on cognitive performance and mood in medical house officers. *British Medical Journal*, **295**, 1513–1516.

Department of Health (1991). *Hours of Work of Doctors in Training: the New Deal*. London: Department of Health.

Doherty, C.C., Stott, G., McCluggage, J.R. and Shanks, R.G. (1992). Educational supervision of pre-registration house officers. *The Ulster Medical Journal*, **61**, 29–34.

Dowling, S. and Barret, S. (1991). *Doctors in the Making: the Experience of the Preregistration Year*. Bristol: SAUS Publications.

Firth-Cozens, J. (1987). Emotional distress in junior house officers. *British Medical Journal*, **295**, 533–535.

Firth-Cozens, J. (1993). Stress, psychological performance and clinical performance. In C. Vincent (Ed.) *Medical Accidents*. Oxford: Oxford University Press.

Firth-Cozens, J. (1997). Predicting stress in general practitioners: 10 year follow up study. *British Medical Journal*, **315**, 34–35.

Firth-Cozens, J. and Greenhalgh, J. (1997). Doctors' perceptions of the links between stress and lowered clinical care. *Social Science and Medicine*, **44**, 1017–1022.

Firth-Cozens, J. and Morrison, L.A. (1989). Sources of stress and ways of coping in junior house officers. *Stress Medicine*, **5**, 121–126.

Friedman, R.C., Bigger, T.J. and Kornfield, D.S. (1971). The intern and sleep loss. *New England Journal of Medicine*, **285**, 201–203.

Gale, R., Jackson, G. and Nicholls, M. (1992). How to run an induction meeting for house officers. *British Medical Journal*, **304**, 1619–1620.

Garrud, P. (1990). Counselling needs and experience of junior hospital doctors. *British Medical Journal*, **300**, 445–447.

General Medical Council (1992). *Tomorrow's Doctors*.

Girard, D.E., Hickham, D.H., Gordon, G.H. and Robison, R.O. (1991). A prospective study of internal medicine residents emotions and attitudes to their training. *Academic Medicine*, **66**, 111–114.

Gottlieb, D.J., Parenti, C., Peterson, C.A. and Lofgren, R.P. (1991). Effect of a change in house staff work schedule on resource utilisation and patient care. *Archives of International Medicine*, **151**, 2065–2070.

Grainger, C., Harries, E., Temple, J. and Griffiths, R. (1996). Junior doctors' job satisfaction and health: changes with seniority. *Health Trends*, **28**, 132–134.

Hale, R. (1998). Doctors in trouble: the MedNet service. In E. Paice (Ed.) *Delivering the New Doctor* (pp. 68–71). Edinburgh: ASME.

Hardy, G., Shapiro, D.A. and Borrill, C.S. (1997). Fatigue in the workforce of the National Health Service Trusts; symptomatology and links with minor psychiatric disorder, demographic, occupational and work role factors. *Journal of Psychosomatic Research*, **43**, 83–92.

Heyworth, J., Whitley, T.W., Allison, E.J. and Revicki, D.A. (1993). Predictors of work satisfaction among SHOs during accident and emergency medicine training. Archives of Emergency Medicine, **10**, 279–288.

NHS Management Executive (1994). *Introduction of Compulsory Induction Courses and Changing the Starting Day for all Hospital and Medical and Dental Staff*, EL(94)1. London: Department of Health.

Jackson, G. (1998). Induction that works: the Lewisham experience. In E. Paice (Ed.) *Delivering the New Doctor* (pp. 40–46) Edinburgh: ASME.

Kiff, R.S. and Sykes, P.A. (1988). Who undertakes consultations in the outpatient department? *British Medical Journal*, **296**, 1511–1512.

King, M.B., Cockcroft, A. and Gooch, C. (1992). Emotional distress: sources, effects and help sought. *Journal of the Royal Society of Medicine*, **85**, 605–608.

Koay, C.B. and Marks, N.J. (1996). A nurse-led pre-admission clinic for elective ENT surgery: the first 8 months. *Annuals of the Royal College of Surgeons, England*, **78**, 15–19.

Lingenfelser, T.H., Kaschel, R., Weber, A., Zaiser-Kaschel, H., Jakober, B. and Kuper, J. (1994). Young hospital doctors after night duty: their task specific cognitive status and emotional condition. *Medical Education*, **28**, 566–572.

McCue, J. (1985). The distress of internship. *New England Journal of Medicine*, **312**, 449–452.

McKee, M. and Black, N. (1992). Does the current use of junior hospital doctors in the United Kingdom affect the quality of medical care? *Social Science and Medicine*, **34**, 549–558.

McKee, M. and Black, N. (1993). Junior doctors work at night: what is done and how much of it is appropriate? *Journal of Public Health Medicine*, **15**, 16–24.

McKevitt, C., Morgan, M., Dundas, R. and Holland, W.W. (1997). Sickness absence and "working through" illness: a comparison of two professional groups. *Journal of Public Health Medicine*, **19**, 295–300.

Masterton, J.P. (1965). Sleep of hospital medical staff. *Lancet*, **ii**, 41–42.

Moss, F. and McManus, I.C. (1992). The anxieties of new clinical students. *Medical Education*, **26**, 17–20.

Moss, F. and Miller, C. (1998). Getting the organisational environment right. In E. Paice (Ed.) *Delivering the New Doctor* (pp. 27–32). Edinburgh: ASME.

Paice, E. (1997). Why do young doctors leave the profession? *Journal of the Royal Society of Medicine*, **90**, 417–418.

Paice, E. (1998). Is the New Deal compatible with good training? A survey of senior house officers. *Hospital Medicine*, **59**, 72–74.

Paice, E. and Craig, G. (1997). *The North Thames Trainees' Point of View Survey*. London: Thames Postgraduate Medical and Dental Education.

Paice, E. and Ingham Clark, C. (1997). *The Hospital at Night*. London: Thames Postgraduate Medical and Dental Education.

Paice, E., Moss, F. and Grant, J. (1997). Association of use of a log book and experience as a pre-registration house officer. *British Medical Journal*, **3**, 213–214.

Paice, E., West, G., Cooper, R., Orton, V. and Scotland A. (1997). Senior house officer training: is it getting better? *British Medical Journal*, **314**, 719–720.

Read, M. and Draycott, T. (1998). Night vision. Can junior doctors be reduced without threatening their training? *Health Service Journal*, January, 24–25.

Richardson, C. (1998). Shadowing: the Leicester experience. In E. Paice (Ed.) *Delivering the New Doctor*. Edinburgh: ASME.

Scott, R.A., Aiken, L.H., Mechanic, D. and Moravsic, J. (1995). Organisational aspects of caring. *The Millbank Quarterly*. **73**, 77–95.

Sutherland, V.J. and Cooper, C.L. (1993). Identifying distress among general practitioners: predictors of psychological ill health and job dissatisfaction. *Social Science Medicine*, **37**, 575–581.

Teahon, K. and Bateman, D.N. (1993). A survey of intravenous drug administration by pre-registration house officers. *British Medical Journal*, **207**, 605–606.

16

DOCTORS IN TROUBLE

Robert Hale and Liam Hudson

This chapter describes a service for "doctors in need of psychological help". It is run by a psychoanalyst, and while offering a broad range of service the fundamental understanding is psychoanalytic. The service is funded by the postgraduate medical dean and is available to all those qualified doctors in our region who are in a training role, whether as trainers or trainees. Individuals come because they recognise that they are in trouble, or because others find their professional behaviour unacceptable and are worried about their mental health—or, of course, a combination of the two. Doctors coming to the service are offered up to six assessment sessions. Should this be required, they are then referred to another agency for further treatment. In the first 22 months since the regional dean took over the funding of the service, 64 doctors were seen. While this chapter concentrates on the treatment of doctors, many of the principles enunciated are applicable to health workers in general.

The overriding principle governing any such service is that of confidentiality. While the postgraduate dean funds the service, neither she nor her staff has access, direct or indirect, to the information it yields about identifiable individuals. There are a few exceptions. These arise when the therapist believes that doctors in treatment may be a danger to their patients. In these cases, and following discussion with the doctors themselves, disclosure may from time to time be necessary. Further, the treatment is offered in an institution both geographically and organisationally separate from the one in which the doctor works, and doctors can use it without fear of being noticed. Shift systems within medicine are a reality, too, and these must be accommodated. To do this runs counter to

Stress in Health Professionals. Edited by Jenny Firth-Cozens and Roy L. Payne
© 1999 John Wiley & Sons Ltd

an important tradition within psychotherapy of consistent and inviolable structure; but compromises must often in practice be struck.

STRESS AND ANXIETY

The terms "stress" and "stress management" are now in general currency, and are valuable as a shorthand for the multiplicity of difficulties, both acknowledged and unacknowledgeable, that can impinge on the individual (O'Leary, 1990; Friedman *et al.*, 1992; Morgan, 1992). Especially influential has been the discovery (Holmes and Rahe, 1967; Brown, 1986) that apparently benign changes (marriage, for instance, or the birth of a child) can exert as much pressure on the physical health and well-being of the individual as the self-evidently distressing (the death of a spouse or a jail sentence). The implication, psychologically speaking, is that stress derives not so much from the noxiousness of a specific stimulus as from the disturbance of equilibrium.

Exclusive reliance on the popularly accepted view of stress can nevertheless be misleading. The implicit metaphor is mechanical, and it misleads in as much as it encourages a purely external view of the difficulties individuals experience. And it also does so if it diverts attention from the personal nature and origins of the vulnerability of those individuals. Sources of stress are both external and internal, institutional and intrapsychic; and these interact (Taylor, 1987; Firth-Cozens, 1992). Sleep deprivation, an institutionally sanctioned stressor routinely experienced by doctors in the course of their training, may exacerbate sources of disturbance which are ingrained features of those doctors' personalities—a chronic lack of self-confidence, say, traceable in turn to the unsatisfactory nature of their ties with their parents.

Both more versatile and less tendentious is the notion of *anxiety*—a state of mind akin to fear. (Anxiety is typically objectless. Fear—the fear of snakes, the fear of failure—in contrast usually has a specific focus.) Learning theory has conventionally accorded anxiety a peripheral role: that of a secondary drive which acts to motivate avoidance of an unpleasant stimulus. Within psychodynamic theory, in contrast, the concept of anxiety is centrally placed; and a distinction is drawn between "primary" anxiety, associated with threats to the system's equilibrium and normally experienced only in nightmares, and "signal" anxiety which alerts the individual to the existence of such threats (Rycroft, 1968). Signal anxiety leads to the adoption of the defensive strategies which enable us to function competently, and it also underlies the formation of those enduring traits, attitudes and beliefs which render us intelligible not just as types but as recognisable individuals. At the heart of such adaptations, in the instance of the doctor, are the choice of a specialty, the development of an appropriate loyalty to it, and a commitment to the distinctive system of values within which medicine is lodged.

INDIVIDUAL DEFENCES

In all fields of medicine, doctors are required to transform the shocking into the mundane; and, in doing so, to contain the unacknowledged anxieties their patients project onto them. In coping, we each rely on defensive structures, institutional and individual, which for the most part serve us well. Some of the self-protective manoeuvres available to the doctor are more obvious than others:

1. We may *deny* that we are experiencing anxiety or tension.
2. We easily become *hypomanic*, workaholic—"riding the tiger", as the saying has it. (He who rides the tiger can't get off because the tiger will eat him.)
3. We *intellectualise*, or "medicalise". We cast a personal problem solely in terms which are logical, controllable.
4. We become *hypochondriacal*. While a neurotic symptom, hypochondria can also serve the anxious doctor as a form of defence. There can be few medical students who have not "had" Hodgkin's disease or leukaemia. The doctor "borrows" his patients' illnesses—the potentially lethal ones especially.
5. Our experience can become *eroticised*. The stuff that medical soaps are made of, an escape into a multiplicity of sexual attractions and encounters may seem to confirm that we are alive and vibrant in the face of depression and physical decay.
6. We may be seized by *black humour*. Magically this transforms the terrifying, sad or disgusting into hilarity. We first encounter it in anatomy dissecting rooms and it often surfaces in the hospital mess or in the pub.
7. We *act out*. We may become medically overactive, giving prescriptions patients do not need, or performing unnecessary operations. We may take addictive drugs or drink excessively or drive too fast. We may also commit suicide. Doctors have high rates of suicide compared with those of other professionals, and this is especially so for those doctors who practise in the United Kingdom but who were trained abroad. (Richings *et al.*, 1986)

This list is by no means exhaustive, of course, but it does refer specifically to the defences which doctors employ. Other professions will employ different defensive structures. We, as doctors, develop our own pattern of defences, their shape determined by the interaction of the personality we bring to medicine with the distinctive anxieties of the branch of medicine in which we specialise. Psychodynamic theory conceives of the individual as an equilibrium-seeking system, within which anxiety causes us to partition experience between the acknowledged and the ignored or denied (Hudson, 1998). From a more specifically psychoanalytic perspective, it is the relationships and experiences of childhood which are seen as the key determinants of such adult adaptations. Not only do these focus the expression of genetic and intrauterine influences, translating them into culturally recognisable forms. They contribute causally in their own right, by establishing—or failing to establish—those primitive bonds of trust between child and parent on which, later in life, resilience to stress is going to depend. There is a further argument, itself psychoanalytic in inspiration (Jaques, 1955; Menzies, 1961), which conceives of institutions—firms, hospitals—as themselves taking on the form they do as a defence against the anxiety and depression of those who work inside them.

In this chapter, two cases are presented. The doctors in question are alike in that the sources of their distress are predominantly internal; the psychological concomitants of developmental crises left unresolved. They differ in that the first doctor is seriously ill whereas the second is not. They also differ culturally, in that the first springs from a background of pronounced cultural fissure and personal dislocation; the second from a background which is altogether more coherent. A plausible reading of the evidence about them is that the fissured background of the first has contributed materially to the severity of her illness, and that the coherence of the second's background has served as a source of psychological strength.

Dr Y

Reluctant to seek help, Dr Y first made contact with the service at the suggestion of a doctor already in treatment. She is aged 40, and works in a relatively small general practice with two other partners and with a list of some 7,000 patients. Depressed, she says that her partners are to some extent aware of the depths of her difficulties and are "very supportive". Her difficulties had seemed to start three years ago, when she realised that a relationship was going to fail. In fact, it ran on for two further years, but eventually broke up. The break-up coincided with the onset of her mother's fatal illness from chronic heart failure. Dr Y now lives with her ageing father. She feels, irrationally, that she precipitated her mother's illness and experiences an overwhelming sense of pointlessness and failure.

She is the youngest of six children, and the only one now unmarried. Her parents came to the UK in 1972; at least in part so that she, the youngest, could have a proper education. Her father and oldest brother urgently wanted her to study medicine, and in doing so she became the family's success story—in her own phrase, its "status symbol". Her mother, on the other hand remained sceptical, hoping that she would become a wife and mother. Dr Y herself, she now claims, entertained doubts. Often she would say to her mother, "I wish I was like you. Uneducated. A mum." In her early twenties, Dr Y entered a marriage which had her family's approval, and went abroad with her new husband. After two years, it was clear that the marriage was not going to succeed, and she decided to end it. Pregnant at the time, and feeling the need to choose between her husband and her unborn child, she had a termination: "I feel now that I'm being punished for what I did then. I feel so guilty about what I did."

Although Dr Y's troubles surfaced in her late thirties, their sources lay in a familiar but in her case unresolved conflict between career and motherhood. Her father had taken one view, her mother another. Where her father wanted her to embrace the values of Western society, her mother remained rooted in those of her more traditional culture—the one within which Dr Y had grown up until she was a teenager, and which embodied strong expectations about the destiny of women as mothers and home-makers. It is one thing for an able teenaged girl to be uprooted from one culture and transplanted to another if both parents adopt similar attitudes towards the move. It is quite another if her mother pulls in one direction and her father in another. In as much as Dr Y could commit herself wholeheartedly to the values and mores of modern Britain, she was severing herself from the assumptive world within which she had grown up and in which her mother remained firmly lodged. Worse, the removal from a traditional culture to a modern culture was one that was to be justified in her father's eyes, in part at least, by her professional success, her future as the family's "status symbol".

The literature on outsiders and emigrés suggests that the removal from one culture to another is often accompanied by a release of imaginative energy and entrepreneurial vigour (Hudson and Jacot, 1986). In Dr Y's case, no such release occurred—presumably because, at some primitive level, her identifications and loyalties were divided. Her career as a doctor was the expression not so much of her own longings but of her father's and eldest brother's longings for her. Not only has she reached the age of 40 as the only member of her family unmarried and childless. There is a sense, it follows, in which she sacrificed her career as a mother to her medical career—a career about which she was bound to be equivocal, and about which she became increasingly uncertain as the pressure exerted on her by her patients mounted. She is aware, now, that she is not investing herself in the practice as she should, and often finds herself resenting the demands her patients make. These she finds trivial. "I feel I'm constantly having to give."

Dr Y's efforts to help herself fluctuate are interspersed with episodes which are openly self-destructive. She has taken three overdoses; tried to strangle herself; and on her fortieth birthday drove up and down the motorway at high speed hoping that someone would cause her to crash. "When you are suicidal, you think of nothing else. Afterwards, it's frightening to realise how crazy you've been."

At the end of the first meeting with her therapist (RH), it was clear that Dr Y needed both immediate support and long-term psychotherapy. With her permission, her GP was contacted—he was the family's doctor but was unaware of her difficulties and had not previously been consulted by her about them. He was asked to prescribe paroxetine, an antidepressant drug, and agreed. Dr Y and her therapist arranged to meet again in three days' time.

Subsequently, Dr Y was to spend a substantial period off work. In a session four months after the first contact, she spoke of the anxieties she had experienced in her first return to general practice. She found herself doubting her own judgement. She said that she had been looking through the notes of cases that she had been dealing with before she had gone sick. There was a woman who had presented with a cough. In the intervening two months the cough had persisted. Dr Y's partner had referred the patient and a carcinoma had been found. Dr Y felt at once that the fault was hers. The therapist pointed out to Dr Y that she was her own harshest critic. Most doctors would have acted as she acted, but would not now feel guilty. Normally, she would have been able to cope. She agreed. "Yes, I would've laughed it off." She went on to describe how her patients were demanding so much of her and how hard she found it. They were waiting for her to come back. Her therapist replied that perhaps they were also telling her that they were angry with her for having gone away in the first place. She said that she couldn't stand up to her patients as she once could. She told of a woman who—yet again—had come in demanding medication that she, Dr Y, knew was unnecessary. In the past Dr Y had stood up to her. Recently the patient had been to see a consultant who had confirmed in a letter that the patient did not need the medication. The patient told Dr Y, nevertheless, that the consultant had said that she should have a small amount of the medication just in case there was a crisis. Dr Y said that she had given in to the patient because she couldn't face an argument. The therapist suggested that she was upset because neither she nor the patient could face the anxiety underlying the patient's insistent request. She knew that the patient's demand expressed her terror of being left without a safety line. In her still fragile state Dr Y realises that her own anxieties are mirrored in those of her patients. As she recovers, she recognises that she must keep separate her patients' unacknowledged terrors from her own.

Dr C

Tall, elegant and trendily dressed, Dr C is for all the world the epitome of the successful young doctor. She comes from a medical family, her cultural background as coherent as Dr Y's is fissured. Despite a rebellious adolescence in which she became a punk, she managed by the time she was 17 to have a choice between art school, music school and medical school. By the time she was 26, she had a first in her BSc, honours in one part of her finals, and had passed both parts of her Membership at first attempt. Now, two years later, she is established in a registrar's post in a top London postgraduate hospital. Unlike Dr Y, she is in no obvious sense ill. Something was nonetheless sufficiently amiss with her life, both professional and private, to bring her into therapy.

The account given here is drawn from a single session, as usual on a Saturday morning. It pays attention to the detail of her exchanges with her therapist:

> DR C: *After I saw you a fortnight ago I felt really pissed off. You made me recognise how hard a time I was giving my boyfriend. I apologised and all he could do was chuck it back in my face. He said he couldn't cope with my moods. He couldn't understand that I was telling him that I recognised how much I loaded onto him. He said he just couldn't cope with me.*

> I said that she must feel angry with me for making her vulnerable. She seemed to be telling me that therapy was removing her defences—an inevitable consequence of therapy in its early stages.

> DR C: *Well, it's been a pretty lousy fortnight anyway. My boss has been away, and there has been this terribly sick woman; we thought she was going to die. The awful thing was that we couldn't find out why. She had septicaemia and we couldn't find the cause. We just had to watch her going down hill. The other consultants came and gave their opinions but they didn't seemed concerned in the way he is. It was all very well for those consultants. She wasn't their patient. They could just walk away from her. On my nights off, I just couldn't sleep.*

> Her last session had evidently shaken her, and I asked why.

DR C: It was realising that I was still the Princess who gets what she wants, and people do what she wants.

I noticed then that she was crying. On the last occasion but one, I reminded her, she had turned up at the clinic, although I had told her well in advance I would be away. Again, I pointed out to her the omnipotent nature of her thought: the assumption that I would be waiting for her, when she knew, consciously, that I was not going to be there. At the time, she had jumped back into her car with a mixture of anger and disappointment and real relief; relief that there were things inside her that she wouldn't have to face.

DR C: You are just not expected to be weak when you are a doctor. The day before yesterday, I was caught in the corridor by the wife of a man who has leukaemia. The consultant was going to tell him at lunch-time, but his wife had already guessed. She was furious with me. Why couldn't I tell her? I had been up all the night before and really couldn't cope with her shouting at me. I didn't handle it at all well. I went to the sluice and locked the door and cried for a bit. Then I realised I had to tell the patient straightaway. As I was going to tell him, his wife came in. I had to tell her to go away. I hated myself for what I was doing because I knew she was so frightened.

I replied that she was telling me about life-shattering events for which she felt responsible and with which she was expected to cope. At the back of her mind, she was uneasy about where her boss had been—and, more importantly, where I had been. I pointed out that she had rung me the previous week to say that she could not make the session because she was still coping with the patients she had admitted the night before. She must feel, somewhere, that I should make time for her in the way that she made time for her patients.

DR C: Yes, but look what it does to you when you really care about your patients. My boss, Brian—he has been a consultant for only two years. He's thirty-nine, but he looks twenty years older. He's balding and going grey.

I made no comment.

DR C: He's the one that everyone wants to refer patients to because he cares. He works morning, noon and night.

I said that she was worried about who looked after Brian, and that she felt responsible for him as well as for her patients.

DR C: Well, I don't want to look after him, and I'm not sure now that I want to be him. The other day, I found myself sitting in the middle of the ward saying out loud "Where am I going", and people said "Now Sarah is really losing her marbles".

I asked how people cope without losing their marbles.

DR C: *Well, most medics do. They can just shut off. They can look at it as an intellectual exercise. Even Brian does that at times. We had a post-mortem over the woman who had just died. We all sat round and talked about the pathology findings. Nobody really talked about what they felt inside.*

I said that I thought she was struggling to find a place where she could talk about these feelings, and that in a way she was bringing the need of her whole unit with her to our sessions.

DR C: *Yes, but that's not much use, because how can I feed it back into them when they can't hear it?*

I said that she was telling me today about the dilemma of being the omnipotent medical Princess yet of having to face the reality that people die and that you can do nothing. Part of her was telling me too that therapy didn't help either. It was the end of the session. She got out her diary, and we made the next appointment, fitting it in with her time off-duty.

The course of psychotherapy is hard to foresee. In the cases of Dr Y and Dr C, the hope is that they will learn to recognise as dysfunctional their own preoccupations and traits: Dr Y's guilt and Dr C's omnipotence. It is also hoped they will learn, in their therapy, to distinguish more clearly between their patients' unacknowledged anxieties and their own. Both may well move within the profession towards niches in which the demands made upon them are more congruous with their own capacities to cope. It could be, for example, that Dr Y will move from general practice and the incessant emotional demands its patients make, into work where contact with patients is more carefully regulated—or even into laboratory research. Dr C could move too. In her case, the prestige of her present position is bound to make a sideways move seem like a defeat; but she could nonetheless switch from physical medicine to a specialty where her psychological sensitivity would become an advantage. She might move, for example, in the direction of psychiatry or pediatrics—or fill Dr Y's place in the ranks of the GPs.

PATIENTS WHO ARE REFERRED

With both Dr Y and Dr C, who had come to the service voluntarily, the enterprise of therapy was collaborative. Unsurprisingly, when approached for permission to publish the clinical material, albeit appropriately disguised, each gave her permission. Unlike them, approximately one third of the doctors seen in the service were referred by their consultant or clinical tutor. Working with doctors who have been referred in this way, the therapist becomes forcefully aware that different anxieties are in play; the doctors' preoccupations often being paranoid in character, and the fantasies those of persecution. Questions of allegiance and absolute confidentiality here become crucial issues; and, for this reason, it was felt inappropriate to present clinical material in this chapter from a doctor who had been referred.

It should be said, nevertheless, that the position of the referred doctor is rarely simple. One doctor may become the focus and scapegoat for a troubled unit or hospital. In effect, doctors may come for therapy on their firm's behalf. Often it takes a crisis, sometimes a crisis with legal implications, for the need—whether individual or collective—to be recognised. For the doctors on whom such pressures play, there is the reasonable fear of being labelled sick, mad, or inadequate—the weak link in a macho team. Small wonder that many doctors, junior or senior, can regard seeking psychological help as tantamount to professional suicide. This is particularly so for those working in the specialties with the highest prestige; and in teams where excellence is sustained on the strength of the prime movers' latent psychopathology.

The position of the referred doctor has a further complication. Often a clash of cultures plays its part in the story, as it did for Dr Y; and with such clashes come the possibility of ethnic or racial prejudice. A feature of the present service bears on this possibility. Nearly three-quarters of the doctors using the service were trained in the UK. Of these, just over half were self-referred, the others being referred either by their consultants or by their clinical tutors. The remaining quarter of the doctors using the service were foreign-trained; and of these, all but three came because they were referred by their consultants or clinical tutors. Many of the home-trained experience themselves as troubled and come for help of their own accord; in other words, this pattern is unusual among the foreign-trained (Hale and Hudson, 1992). The consequence is that many of those foreign-trained doctors who use the service do so seized with thoughts of rejection and persecution which obstruct the development of a collaborative atmosphere. Regrettably, then, the experience of collaborative therapy within the service is at present very largely restricted to work with doctors trained in the UK.

A FINAL THOUGHT

Our hospitals grew out of institutions which were religious in nature, informed by religious values. Altruism remains central to the practice of medicine in the British Isles to this day. Recently, however, new and more commercial values have been introduced. A small but significant proportion of the doctors who refer themselves to the service as patients do so as a result of these changes. Typically, their firms are experiencing difficulty in meeting financial targets; a constraint which is not only unfamiliar but which seems to violate the doctors' ethic of care. Usually it is the consultant who comes on these grounds; but more than once it has been a junior doctor who comes, as it were, as emissary.

The new ways of the Health Service undermine the existing defences of many doctors, and do so both at a personal level and at the level of the institution. Many of the pressures exerted are indiscriminate, causing anxiety in the minds of the more and less dedicated alike. They may also be gratuitous in that, with appropriate care, their effect could be mitigated or avoided altogether. It may not be unduly difficult to design forms of medical training which preserve the doctor's traditional altruism, but which at the same time acknowledge the severity of the psychological demands which the practice of medicine in a cost-conscious Health Service can make.

REFERENCES

Brown, R. (1986). *Social Psychology, the Second Edition* (pp. 635–685) London: Collier Macmillan.

Friedman, E.S., Clark, D.B. and Gershon, S. (1992). Stress, anxiety and depression. *Journal of Anxiety Disorders*, **6**, 337–363.

Firth-Cozens, J. (1992). The role of early family experiences in the perception of organizational stress. *Journal of Occupational and Organizational Psychology*, **65**, 61–75.

Hale, R. and Hudson, L. (1992). The Tavistock study of young doctors. *British Journal of Hospital Medicine*, **47**, 452–464.

Holmes, T.H. and Rahe, R.H. (1967). The social readjustment rating scale. *Journal of Psychosomatic Research*, **11**, 213–218.

Hudson, L. (1998). *Strangely Familiar: The Psychological Significance of Boundaries and of What Lies Beyond Them.* Tanner Lecture on Human Values, Yale University, 14 April, 1997, Salt Lake City: University of Utah Press.

Hudson, L. and Jacot, B. (1986). The outsider in science. In C. Bagley and G.K.Verma (Eds) *Personality, Cognition and Values.* London: Macmillan.

Jaques, E. (1955). Social systems as a defence against persecutory and depressive anxiety. In M. Klein, P. Helmann and R.E. Money-Kyrle (Eds) *New Directions in Psychoanalysis.* London: Tavistock.

Menzies, I.E.P. (1961). *The Functioning of Social Systems as a Defence against Anxiety.* Tavistock Pamphlet No. 3. London: Tavistock.

Morgan, D.R. (Ed.) (1992). *Stress and the Medical Profession.* London: British Medical Association.

O'Leary, A. (1990). Stress, emotion, and human immune function. *Psychological Bulletin*, **108**, 363–382.

Rycroft, C. (1968). *Anxiety and Neurosis*. Harmondsworth: Penguin.
Richings, J.C., Khara, G.S. and McDowell, M. (1986). Suicide in young doctors. *British Journal of Psychiatry*, **149**, 475–478.
Taylor, G.J. (1987). *Psychosomatic Medicine and Contemporary Psychoanalysis*. Madison, CT: International Universities Press.

17

SETTING UP A WORKPLACE COUNSELLING SERVICE

Til Wykes and Richard Whittington

INTRODUCTION

Workplace stress is acknowledged to be an important factor not only in the quality of the delivery of care but also in recruitment, absenteeism and turnover of highly trained staff. Staff in the USA have become particularly litigious in suing their employers for the health damage produced by stressors at work. In 1994, in the UK, Mr Justice Colman ruled that employers had a common law duty to provide a safe environment and that this included assessing the risk to mental health by stress experienced at work.

The mental health of the workforce of the UK National Health Service (NHS) has been identified as a high priority in several recent policy pronouncements (Department of Health, 1997a, 1997b; Cockcroft and Williams, 1998). In particular the 1998 Green Paper, *Our Healthier Nation*, recognises that the NHS, as the largest British employer, has a responsibility to set an example in terms of promoting mental health among the workforce (Department of Health, 1998). But although there is a recognition of the importance of workplace stress, it is still not clear what this will mean in practice. How will these policy commitments be translated into effective interventions?

Stress in Health Professionals. Edited by Jenny Firth-Cozens and Roy L. Payne
© 1999 John Wiley & Sons Ltd

One possible intervention is to set up workplace counselling schemes, but these must be seen in the context of other sorts of interventions which may also reduce the problems of workplace stress. In this chapter we will consider some of the options in addition to workplace counselling services as well as the remit for the counselling service itself.

PRINCIPLES OF WORKPLACE STRESS INTERVENTIONS

Well-planned interventions must be based on an awareness of the types of demands faced by staff and the "locus of control" of workplace stress. As other chapters demonstrate, health care staff report relatively high levels of psychological stress and face a broad range of demands in their work. These stressors can be either chronic and endemic to the job or acute. The usual response to the question about "What sort of interventions should be available?" is to provide individual counselling services. They fit well into the philosophy that stress is an employee problem, not a management problem and they do not involve major structural or functional changes in the organisation.

Nevertheless, we do know that organisational interventions can decrease employee stress (see Murphy in Chapter 11 and Ivancevich et al., 1990, for a review) even if the maintenance of benefits of these changes has not been established. Our view is that the primary concern of any intervention should be with stressor reduction. This implies that organisational changes, particularly in the management of the workforce, are required and certainly several researchers have highlighted this area (e.g. Carson et al., 1995; Thomas, 1997). But some of these interventions are also important in the context of workplace counselling. In fact, without the organisation being seen to be auditing stress and trying to make changes which reduce stressors, any other interventions at the individual level may be seen as making the workforce totally responsible for its own stress.

PREVENTION VS TREATMENT

A fundamental issue in any aspect of a health care problem is to consider treatment as secondary to prevention in terms of priorities. Clearly, one extremely controversial way of preventing severe stress responses would be to screen the workforce to identify individuals at risk. This is clearly not a feasible option although Firth-Cozens (1997) has argued that an identification process for the purpose of the intervention could be carried out at the stage of professional education. However, in order for such an intervention to be acceptable there needs to be a commitment from senior staff and credibility for such a policy to be established with managers, employees and trade unions.

Alternative interventions at the organisational level include alleviating stressors by various forms of stress management. These include not only traditional stress management interventions but also staff support groups. These groups have been available in some healthcare settings since the 1980s and their value, if used correctly, is well known (Carson *et al.*, 1995).

EFFECTIVENESS OF INTERVENTIONS

Research on workplace counselling, such as employee assistance schemes, has suggested that they save organisations hard cash. For example, in the USA the Department of Health and Human Services Counselling Services was evaluated (Maiden, 1988). Over the 30 months of the evaluation the service saw 2,500 staff. The control group comprised those who worked in the same health service but who did not attend the counselling service. The results showed that for every dollar spent on counselling about seven dollars were saved. In the UK there is also evidence that workplace counselling can be beneficial for the people who are referred. For example, in an uncontrolled study Mitchie (1996) found that short-term counselling interventions with health care staff not only affected positively people's mood at post-treatment and follow up, but also reduced absenteeism. Highley-Marchington and Cooper (1997), in a study of three EAPs, have also reported that individual counselling affects both psychological well-being and absence in those who were counselled. However, in their study there was no effect of the provision of a counselling service on other staff who were not counselled. In other words, in order to get a change at the organisational level, an organisational rather than an individual level change must be instigated.

There are, of course, problems with the evaluation of workplace counselling, as the next chapter describes in detail. Many studies do not employ a comparison group, which is essential, but the choice of an appropriate one is difficult to assess. Also, those staff who contact a counselling service are likely to be exhibiting extreme stress reactions. Finally, when the focus is on workplace counselling the employees' perceptions of their employer may change, and this may also have an effect on organisational activities that are beneficial. This is clearly a result of workplace counselling, but it is not the direct effect which the evaluators are generally searching for.

Reynolds (1997) compared individual counselling with an intervention which increased employees' participation and control. The results indicated that counselling had clear benefits for the counselled employee's psychological wellbeing. Neither intervention, however, had an effect on work characteristics, physical symptoms or absence. Individual interventions that treat existing psychological problems or help employees manage difficult working conditions appear to be better in their efficacy and efficiency.

SPECIAL CONSIDERATION FOR HEALTH SERVICE STAFF?

Some have argued that the health services staff are different from those in other public and private sector organisations. They are costly to train, consume vast resources, and their behaviour affects patient safety. These factors lead to the conclusion that health care professionals need specially tailored workplace stress interventions (Orton, 1996). But most of the factors identified by Orton (1996) are not unique to health care professionals (cf. air traffic controllers). What is unique is their professional self-image as carers of other people. This self-image can lead to a denial of stress problems initially, then heightened distress once control has been lost. For example, many of the staff victims of patient violence identified in a series of studies by Wykes and Whittington (1991, 1998) showed that staff, while denying that they were affected by the incident, were extremely anxious and distressed.

In terms of what is currently available, Payne (1998) cites a Health Education Authority survey of 115 health service trusts and health authorities. Three quarters of these organisations offer some form of counselling and about one-third provided brief stress management interventions. Half the organisations had audited stress levels among their staff, although 80% had no stress management policy or strategy. While all trusts have occupational health departments attached to them, the traditional role of these departments is to treat physical workplace illness and injury. Their ability and willingness to offer expert prevention and treatment of psychological problems is debatable. Counselling services are often found situated within the Occupational Health Department and it is important to identify the different responsibilities of each of these complementary services.

ISSUES IN SETTING UP A WORKPLACE COUNSELLING SERVICE

Why is the organisation providing counselling services?

First there is a legal "duty of care" on employers for their employees' physical, psychological and social well-being. In Britain this is laid out both in statute and in common law. Second, the organisation may decide to include the role of caring for staff as part of its mission statement. Finally, the organisation may provide a service for dealing with an individual's problems because they believe that it will benefit not only the individual's work quality but also the organisation's financial status.

It must be clear from the planning stage of any counselling service which, if any, of these three the counselling service should fulfil. This is important because it not only defines the extent of the service and the skills of the providers of that service but it also outlines the measures of success of such a service.

We have already discussed the problems of identifying organisational benefits from personal counselling. There are benefits for the individuals who access a service but generally the only way to improve the organisation is to carry out organisational change.

A separate service or can managers do it?

Some health services have suggested that staff within the service—that is, managers—can provide an effective service. But it is the view of several researchers (e.g. Martin,1997) that the roles of a counsellor and a manager are incompatible. The duty of managers is to the organisation and, although the skills of counselling may be extremely useful to managers in their appraisal and mentoring of employees, it is not thought that this form of help and guidance can substitute for professional counselling.

Internal vs external services: the pros and cons

Counselling services can be set up in two main ways: in-house counselling provision and out-house (external) provision. There are no substantial empirical data on the outcome of each type of service, although there are proponents of both. For example, Summerfield and Van Oudtshoorn (1995) are in favour of in-house counselling and Highley-Marchington and Cooper (1997) have shown that internal services are more successful than external services in reducing employees' stress. The support for external provision often centres on the issue of confidentiality of the service—an issue that is discussed in more detail later. It is perhaps best not to juxtapose the two types of counselling but to consider the benefits of each. Table 17.1 gives the main benefits as well as some of their drawbacks. These benefits and drawbacks may change depending not only on the type of organisation for which the services are being offered but also on the current position of the organisation. The two sorts of provision can, of course, be combined to provide the best from both systems.

Table 17.1:   The advantages and disadvantages of in-house and external counselling provision

In-house provision	External provision
Benefits	*Benefits*
• The counsellor can be in touch with the organisation	• It can offer clear confidentiality
• The councillor is visible in the organisation	• It can provide a range of services
• The counsellor can provide multiple roles	• It is not reliant on a single provider but can offer a range of counselling skills from a number of providers
• The counsellor can access other informal and formal supports within the organisation	• It is distinct from the organisation
Drawbacks	*Drawbacks*
• More difficult to maintain confidentiality	• The service has to make a profit
• The counsellor is involved with the politics of management	• Counsellor may not know the culture of the organisation
• Counsellor may be strongly identified with either management or staff	• May be seen as an outsider by both clients and management

External services are usually delivered by Employee Assistance Programmes (EAPs) and have developed differently in the UK and the USA. In both countries there is a tendency to use the telephone as a means of communication. In the USA it is used as a means of initial contact and as a clearing house, whereas in the UK it is also used as a means of providing counselling. In the UK this means that there is an immediate availability of different sources of help, from money management to trauma counselling, so that a wide variety of needs can be catered for. In addition to these services, many services also have available a network of counsellors. The essence of their success is the contacts which they develop within an organisation so that they can pass on contextual information to the counsellors dealing with that organisation. EAPs can tailor their services to the demands of the organisation and be flexible.

Confidentiality: ethical issues

The usual argument for external counselling provision is to ensure confidentiality. But confidentiality is a matter of perception rather than a reality, and it is obvious that external services may have an easier time persuading their clients of complete confidentiality than internal services. This is not to say that those which are internal cannot provide a service which is beyond reproach; rather, that it is more difficult for them to illustrate this aspect of their service. Clearly, all counselling services within organisations must provide some information to managers on the use of the service, and the employer also has the right to expect that it could be audited for its effectiveness.

Confidentiality is not only defined by the leakage of information between the employer and the counsellor but also in the visibility of the service. An employee's willingness to use a counselling service at work is clearly affected by whether he or she thinks that the use of a service will be visible.

All counsellors should be governed by some ethical principles from a professional organisation (e.g. British Psychological Society, British Association of Counselling, United Kingdom Council for Psychotherapy). Membership of appropriate bodies often occurs when counsellors are employed as part of the health services, but is rarer in commercial organisations. These professional organisations prescribe similar professional codes of conduct which are relatively easy to follow, and define specific procedures which should be implemented in problematic situations. But the workplace will also have expectations about what information it wishes to be disclosed and this may not be completely obvious when a counselling service is commenced. Ethical guidelines for counselling within organisations are not well developed but there are a few points which an organisation must bear in mind when drawing up its counselling contract. They are drawn from Shea and Bond (1997) and Bond (1993) who should be read in more detail by both counsellors and contract managers.

Who is the client?
The relationship is three-way (client–counsellor–organisation) when it is clear that the counselling services are paid for by the organisation, but the primary responsibility of a therapeutic counsellor is owed to the individual who seeks help. This is now established in law. There are, however, some organisational issues, particularly for the health services, which may constrain this principle. This is where the health of patients or other staff may be placed at risk.

Autonomy of the client
The importance of the client's willingness to take part in counselling is extremely high. A workplace can sometimes insist on a member of staff attending counselling, but the counsellor has to allow clients to decide for

themselves whether to take advantage of it. It has to be recognised by the workplace that the employee is autonomous in this matter.

Confidentiality

Information of a personal nature, irrespective of whether it is advantageous or disadvantageous, must only be given with the client's consent. This can be made clear in the counselling contract or negotiated for specific circumstances. Information may also be shared within a team of counsellors or at the very least with a supervisor.

All these principles need to be acknowledged in the form of contract for counselling services, even if the service is provided in-house. In this latter case the issue of the personal contract of employment needs to be considered as well as issues such as record keeping, internal complaints procedure, etc.

DIFFERENCES BETWEEN COUNSELLING AND WORKPLACE COUNSELLING

With the increase in the provision of counselling at work, counsellors have begun to view this area as an employment opportunity on the same level as private individual counselling. Table 17.2 lists the skills required of a workplace counsellor.

Unfortunately, employers are likely to be more impressed by the knowledge that the counsellor may have about the workplace rather than the other skills in the list. Fisher (1997) suggests that it is important to have someone who knows about the context of the NHS, particularly because of the recent changes in its structure. She suggests that counsellors should also have experience in a workplace setting because they then understand the conflicts which arise at the individual/organisation interface.

THE COUNSELLING SYSTEM

By phone or in person?

Some counselling services have initial counselling by phone which allows a number of different counsellors to be available for particular problems. For some health service providers this may prove to be too costly although there have recently been contracts between a number of similar providers who all contribute to the purchase of a broader scheme while still retaining some in-house service. It would certainly be possible for several organisations to negotiate such a scheme.

Table 17.2:   The skills and qualities for a workplace counsellor (adapted from Megranahan, 1989)

Organisational skills	• For understanding the organisational dynamics; for preventing friction between multiple roles; to conduct programme evaluation; to develop company and programme policies; for working out how to publicise the service
Personal qualities	• Assertiveness—to ensure a high profile for the service • Good interpersonal skills—to facilitate the establishment of personal contacts with key personnel
Administrative ability	• Writing skills, ability to produce clear written information about the service, brochures policy statements, etc. • Personal time management and organisational skills
Additional skills	• Knowledge of professional ethics • Financial counselling skills • Knowledge of legal and illegal drugs • Consultative skills • Training and public-speaking ability
Familiar with	• Organisational structure, job descriptions, job performance expectations and the disciplinary process • Industrial relations and union representation • Benefits package for employees • Social service agencies and health care systems

Time limits on therapy

Because of the workload and likely resource implications, organisations want to employ counsellors to provide a short-term focused approach which is limited in the amount of time allocated to each client. This ensures a throughput of clients and short waiting times. It also ensures that the counsellor can allocate time for crisis management which may be required from time to time. There is evidence that short-term therapy does work in reducing distress and in reducing absenteeism (Mitchie, 1996), although there is still some controversy about its longer term benefits.

Self-referral

Organisations often think that, by employing a counselling service, problem personnel can be immediately referred and the manager's responsibility for the mental health of that member of staff is then transferred. Referral by managers can be counter-productive for any counselling intervention, especially if it carries with it the implicit threats about promotion prospects, continued employment or pay increases. Some services have stopped all management referrals, preferring a sole self-referral process, although this too has its drawbacks. Some staff may seek to be equally coercive in using the counselling process to further their own aims. As a rule, self-referral should be encouraged; however, management referral may be justifiable in some instances where termination of employment or suspension are the only other alternatives.

In order to help the referral system it may be necessary to prompt both the workforce and managers about who should be referred. This then defines the boundaries of workplace counselling. Megranahan (1989) lists the likely psychological states—mainly depression, anxiety and anger—which should result in a referral. But other organisational issues such as regular absences or sicknesses, poor appraisal, anxiety related to specific events such as departmental meetings or presentations and, of course, redundancy can all be dealt with in the workplace counselling service. External events which can also affect work performance—such as bereavement, domestic relationships, alcoholism, and subclinical states such as irritability and moodiness—can also be appropriately referred. One of the obstacles to referral in the health services is the organisational culture. Health service professionals have a very definite view of mental ill-health—it is something that patients have, not the staff. This same "macho" attitude can also result in blame or censure from the staff group of the individual in counselling. This work context has to be considered both for the individual in counselling and in trying to reduce the barriers to initial referral.

DEMANDS ON COUNSELLING STAFF

When starting a counselling service there is great pressure from the organisation to establish the service quickly. If this is not well managed with clear steps then it can lead to dramatic workloads and high expectations from the organisation for the short term. This can lead to burnout of the workplace counsellors themselves. It is also tempting for the counselling service staff to engage in activities that are beyond their skills and training (Roman *et al.*, 1987) particularly when staffing is low. A management plan with clear time-limited expectations is essential to the success of the service. When the service is operating it is important to have a monitoring system in place so that counsellors are not overwhelmed by unrealistic case loads.

Supervision of counselling

Counsellors are required to have supervision from an external source to provide an overview of their work. It is essential that this part of the service is recognised as a cost at the outset and that it is not appropriate for counsellors to be supervised by their line manager. A counsellor may already have supervision arrangements in place which could be continued but the organisation must ensure that this is appropriate for the role of a workplace counsellor.

Publicising counselling

There is little point in having a counselling service if it is not known to employees. Employees are often suspicious of personal counselling, and portraying a positive image at the outset is seen as essential. There are three obvious things employees need to know: that a counselling service exists, how it can be accessed, and what it provides.

Evaluating counselling

As with all interventions within the health service, they must be shown to be effective. This means that data need to be gathered and analysed on key aspects which are thought to measure good outcomes. These might include an anonymous questionnaire asking past clients for their view of the service, carrying out pre- and post-evaluations of psychological distress, as well as broad data such as level of referral and the main characteristics of the referral. These latter will clearly be couched in broad terms so that individual problems are not identified. So, in setting up a counselling service an effective record-keeping system must be established that provides reliable information. The workplace may also want to establish some cost-effectiveness data, although this can be difficult to ascertain. However, it may be possible to establish the effects on absence rates (e.g. Mitchie, 1996).

SETTING UP THE SERVICE

The following list indicates the steps which must be followed if a successful workplace counselling service is to be set up. This list is based on learning from the mistakes of the recent past, particularly from those counselling services within the NHS.

- Identify the needs of staff and the organisation.
- Define the role of the service within the organisation.

- Define the rationale for the service.
- Compare the service costs of various strategies (internal vs external, etc.)
- Agree service.
- Obtain backing of key people and groups within the organisation (managers, trade unions, etc.).
- Clarify the relationship with other services, e.g. occupational health, to prevent role ambiguity.
- Establish guidelines for access to the service (self-referral, management referral, etc.).
- Establish lines of accountability.
- Establish boundaries of confidentiality.
- Draw up clear guidelines on confidentiality and the contract between the counsellor and client.
- Devise methods of data collection and record keeping.
- Ensure a confidential location for counselling.
- Establish an ongoing strategy for publicising the service.
- Identify a local referral network.
- Agree a number of sessions.
- Establish administrative support.
- Agree hours of service availability.
- Provide external clinical supervision.
- Ensure that counsellors have professional indemnity insurance.
- Establish quality assurance system.
- Evaluate the service.

DEVELOPING THE SERVICE

At the beginning there are a number of issues which must be dealt with by the counsellor and/or counselling service. It is important to know, for instance, what is actually wanted from the service which is often not stated overtly. Questions to ask might include:

- Who or what has driven the initiative to set up a workplace counselling service?
- What do senior managers want from the service?
- What do employees want from the service?
- What are the priorities of the interest groups (individuals, senior managers, human resource department)?

With an understanding of these organisational constraints, the service can develop further and move on from purely client work to include staff training, stress management and organisational development. But with these changes may come difficulties, particularly if the counsellor has to deal with clients who are currently in counselling. This can clearly affect the individual client work and affect the confidentiality of the counselling service adversely, and these risks must be taken into account when deciding how to develop the service.

Risks for the counsellor

The service must be prominent or employees will not know how and why to access it. But there are risks in having a high profile. Both managers and employees have expectations that such a service could be used politically to develop their own goals. Sometimes counselled staff wish the workplace counselling service to "put their case to management" and, on the other hand, managers may think that the counselling service is there to "counsel people out of the organisation". Fisher (1997) reports that counsellors in her study were careful about the organisational meetings they attended. This was to prevent them from being too highly associated with either the employer or the staff group.

CONCLUSION

In this chapter we have considered some of the principles underpinning workplace stress interventions and some of the practical issues to be addressed by organisations implementing such approaches. The evidence of high levels of distress among health care staff clearly indicates a general need for support in dealing with a huge range of demands and in many cases a more specific need for focused intervention. There is now a policy commitment for the NHS to become a "good employer" in terms of reducing staff stress, and we have seen some examples of imaginative and effective interventions. Perhaps the greatest hurdle to overcome now is the attitude of the health care staff themselves to the image of the "wounded healer", and how this vulnerable role conflicts with professional and personal identities.

REFERENCES

Bond T. (1993). *Standards and Ethics for Counselling in Action*. London: Sage.
Carroll, M. (1996). *Workplace Counselling: A Systematic Approach to Employee Care*. London: Sage.
Carson, J., Fagin, L. & Ritter, S. (Eds) (1995). *Stress and Coping in Mental Health Nursing*. London: Chapman & Hall.

Cockcroft, A. and Williams, S. (1998). The "New NHS". Staff in the NHS. *British Medical Journal*, **316**, 378.

Dawson, J., Johnson, M., Kehiayan, N., Kyanco, S. and Martinel, R. (1988). Response to patient assault: a peer support programme for nurses. *Journal of Psychosocial and Mental Health Services*, **26**(2), 8–15.

Department of Health (1997a). *Research and Development: Towards an Evidence-based Service*. London: NHS Executive.

Department of Health (1997b). *The New NHS*. London: Department of Health.

Department of Health (1998). *Our Healthier Nation: A Contract for Health*. Consultation Paper. London: HMSO.

Engel, F. and Marsh, S. (1986). Helping the employee victim of violence in hospitals. *Hospital and Community Psychiatry*, **37**, 159–162.

Firth-Cozens, J. (1997). Predicting stress in general practice: ten year follow-up postal survey. *British Medical Journal*, **315**, 34–35.

Fisher, H. (1997). Plastering over the cracks? A study of employee counselling in the NHS. In M. Walton and M. Carroll (Eds) *Handbook of Counselling in Organizations*. London: Sage.

Flannery, R., Fulton, P., Tausch, J. and Deloffi, A. (1991). A programme to help staff cope with the psychological sequelae of assaults by patients. *Hospital and Community Psychiatry*, **42**, 935–938.

Highley-Marchington, C. and Cooper, C. (1997). An evaluation of employee assistance workplace counselling programmes in the UK, in M. Walton and M. Carroll (Eds) *Handbook of Counselling in Organizations*. London: Sage.

Ivancevich, J.M., Matteson, M., Freedman, S. and Phillips, J. (1990). Worksite stress management interventions. *American Psychologist*, **45**, 252–61.

Maiden, R. (1988). EAP evaluation in a Federal Government Agency. *Employee Assistance Quarterly*, **3**, 191–203.

Martin, P. (1997). Counselling skills training for managers in the public sector. In M. Walton and M. Carroll (Eds) *Handbook of Counselling in Organizations*, London: Sage.

Megranahan, P. (1989) *Counselling: A Practical Guide for Employers*. London: Institute of Personnel Management.

Mitchie, S. (1996). Reducing absenteeism by stress management: valuation of a stress counselling service. *Work and Stress*, **10**, 367–372.

Morrison, E. (1988). The assaulted nurse: strategies for healing. *Perspectives in Psychiatric Care*, **24**, 120–126.

Orton, P. (1996). Stress in health care professionals. *British Journal of Health Care Management*, **2**, 91–94.

Payne, D. (1998). Calming measures. *Nursing Times*, **94**(8), 14–15.

Reynolds, S. (1997). Psychological well-being at work: is prevention better than cure? *Journal of Psychosomatic Research*, **43**, 93–102.

Roman, P., Blum, T. and Bennett, N. (1987). Educating organisational consumers about employee assistance programs. *Public Personnel Management*, **16**(4), 299–312.

Shea, C. and Bond, T. (1997). Ethical issues for counselling in organizations. In M. Walton and M. Carroll (Eds) *Handbook of Counselling in Organizations*. London: Sage.

Summerfield, J. and Van Oudtshoorn, L. (1995). *Counselling in the Workplace*. London: Institute of Personnel and Development.

Tehrani, N. (1997). Internal counselling provision for organizations. In M. Walton and M. Carroll (Eds) *Handbook of Counselling in Organizations*. London: Sage.

Thomas, B. (1997). Management strategies to tackle stress in mental health nursing. *Mental Health Care*, **1**, 15–17.

Wykes, T. and Mezey, G. (1994). Counselling for victims of violence. In T. Wykes (Ed.) *Violence and Health Care Professionals*. London: Chapman & Hall.

Wykes, T. and Whittington, R. (1991). Coping strategies used by staff following assault by a patient: an exploratory study. *Work and Stress*, **5**, 37–48.

Wykes, T. and Whittington, R. (1998). Prevalence and predictors of early traumatic stress reactions in assaulted psychiatric nurses. *Journal of Forensic Psychiatry*, **9**, 37–48.

18

PSYCHOTHERAPEUTIC INTERVENTIONS FOR WORK STRESS

Gillian E. Hardy and Michael Barkham

Stress management interventions sit between clinical and occupational psychology theories and practice. In this chapter we discuss the advantages and disadvantages of being able to draw from two distinct strands of psychology. We review the evidence for the effectiveness of psychotherapeutic interventions in reducing work stress from both mental health and worksite perspectives, and discuss three issues that indicate that the research findings from the clinical literature are insufficient to establish psychological interventions as the treatment of choice for stress at work.

There is good evidence, gathered over the past 20 years, to show that psychotherapy is effective for the treatment of depression and anxiety, the two most common minor psychiatric complaints (Roth and Fonagy, 1996). Some of these studies have used work-based measures as indicators of improvement (Barkham and Shapiro, 1990; Elkin *et al.*, 1989; Firth and Shapiro, 1986). Again, the evidence shows that psychotherapeutic interventions are helpful in ameliorating work difficulties, although change in work behaviours and attitudes may happen more slowly than symptom and mood indicators (Mintz *et al.*, 1992). Although many of the studies that have assessed the value of counselling and other psychotherapeutic interventions for work problems are methodologically flawed

---

Stress in Health Professionals. Edited by Jenny Firth-Cozens and Roy L. Payne
© 1999 John Wiley & Sons Ltd

(Berridge and Cooper, 1993; Reynolds and Shapiro, 1991), there is a little, but nevertheless consistent, evidence that counselling offered at the workplace can help individuals who are distressed (Cooper and Sadri, 1991; Ganster *et al.*, 1982).

THREE ISSUES: PROBLEM DEFINITION, CAUSATION, AND ALTERNATIVE INTERVENTIONS

There are three related issues that expose the limitations of existing understandings. The first issue concerns the question of problem definition. What is it that is being targeted for change? Is it mood, behaviour, work-related competencies and skills, interpersonal skills (at work), or organisational indices such as absence or turnover rates, performance and quality? Alternatively, should the goals of an intervention be determined privately between an employee and counsellor or trainer? The arguments generally used to convince managers of the value of having a counselling service available to employees are (a) that employers have a responsibility to protect their staff from harm and (b) that mentally healthy organisations are more productive (Cooper and Cartwright, 1994). The first argument suggests that there are stressors within organisations that can (and should) be minimised and that staff can be trained to recognise these stressors and develop skills to cope with them. The second argument suggests that important outcomes from psychotherapeutic interventions are cost savings and increased productivity. Both arguments indicate that organisations are active in causing stress and can benefit from reductions in levels of stress. Here, then, the outcomes of interventions are not individual, personal goals, but public, measurable organisational targets.

The second issue stems from the first: to agree targets for change demands an understanding of the problem and clarity about the model of causation that will be used to guide interventions. General models of stress focus on individual, internal responses to external stressors (Fisher, 1986). Such interactional models have been adopted in the work stress literature. Three sets of variables are considered: the external work stressors, individual factors (such as Type A personality—Rosenman and Chesney, 1985; or hardiness—Kobasa *et al.*, 1982) and indices of strain (behavioural, cognitive and emotional). These consequences of stress have been linked to the development of illnesses, such as coronary heart disease and gastrointestinal problems, though our understanding of the links between stress and illness is still in its infancy. Nevertheless, methods that have been developed to reduce occupational stress have come primarily from the clinical field using a medical or disease model.

Such models have value: they give a legitimacy, status and power that is conferred on the medical profession. But they reduce the importance of the organisational component of stress models and, as a consequence, reduce the power of stress counsellors or trainers within organisations.

The final issue takes the models of work stress and asks: "Are there better ways of effecting change?" and "What is the appropriate comparison group or intervention?" These issues are concerned with methodological rigour, but are also of theoretical and practical importance. Psychotherapeutic approaches emphasise individual factors over organisational factors, which restricts the development of different interventions (Ganster *et al.*, 1982; Reynolds and Shapiro, 1991). In this chapter we will not discuss alternative approaches to the management of stress, but it is important to recognise that alternative interventions based on different models may be as effective, or more effective, than individual, disease-based approaches.

DEFINITIONS AND DESCRIPTIONS

Psychotherapeutic interventions are generally offered either in a form of prevention (stress management training; SMT), or treatment (counselling). These are generally offered to any member of an organisation, or to groups of staff within the organisation such as specific wards or occupational groups. Only a proportion of staff at SMT is likely to be stressed, and attendance at the training session is rarely dependent on observable signs of strain. For the majority of participants the main aim of the workshop will be to learn how to prevent and better cope with stress. This form of intervention has been described as "re-active prevention" or activities which attempt to improve coping resources before or following exposure to stressful events (Reynolds and Shapiro, 1991). Access to a counsellor, on the other hand, usually requires an individual to show signs of stress or psychological distress. The outcomes of SMT (stress recognition and prevention) and counselling (treatment) are therefore different, although evaluations usually use the same measures for both types of intervention.

STRESS MANAGEMENT TRAINING

SMT is typically offered to groups of staff in anything ranging from one-hour sessions to 20-week courses. Programmes vary, but generally contain an educative component, training in some method of relaxation, self-evaluation and goal setting and related skills training such as assertion skills, time management and problem solving. For example, a typical stress management course would begin with a presentation of a model of occupational stress; the nature, signs, causes and symptoms of stress are described and discussed. Participants often complete "stress inventories" which provide feedback about each person's stress level and potential worksite stressors. Other teaching sessions may include topics such as coping styles, common interpersonal problems and time management. Action planning is usually integral to the courses and participants are encouraged to find ways of support for following through their action plans.

The theoretical models of most programmes are rather loosely based on the person–environment fit model (Caplan et al., 1975). This model emphasises the matching or fit between a person's resources or abilities with the demands of the environment or potential work stressors (such as workload, role conflict and responsibility for others). The usual assumption of individually tailored interventions based on such a model is that increasing a person's knowledge and skills will offset the impact of stressors in the workplace through improved coping resources. As a result many of the techniques used to effect change are based on personality and coping models. For example, participants are often encouraged to evaluate their cognitive style through understanding the attributions they make about stressful events. Participants are generally encouraged to develop active coping behaviours as a way of reducing the impact of potential stressors, i.e. to make changes to their environment as well as to themselves.

Within the literature, no standard or manualised SMT programme has been developed. This means that it is impossible with most studies to examine what are the important components of the programme that help participants, and usually means that each programme is unique and cannot be replicated in future studies. The main reason for this is that most evaluations are of SMT programmes being conducted by practitioners within organisations whose primary goal is to provide a service to that organisation rather than to research. Such work is necessary, but limits the development of improved interventions and understandings of what might be the important techniques that produce change.

Evaluations of these programmes, although often methodologically poor (Auerbach, 1989; Beehr and O'Hara, 1987), generally show some improvement in self-reported psychological symptoms (Sallis et al., 1987), although little change in job-related attitudes (Everly, 1989). Reductions in stress-related symptoms, however, appear to be short lived (Ivancevich et al., 1990), and SMT programmes have been found to have little impact on organisational levels of stress (Murphy, 1996). One exception to this is a study by Jones and colleagues (1988). An intervention that comprised a number of different components (i.e. communication of the results of a stress survey, policy and procedure changes aimed at improving communication, the setting up of an employment assistance programme (EAP)) was found to reduce the frequency of medication errors by 50% in one hospital site, and reduce the number of malpractice claims in another group of hospitals.

There are few systematic comparisons of different stress management packages. One study compared the effectiveness of SMT programmes in three domains: controlling one's physiological reactions (relaxation, nutrition and exercise programmes); skills for coping with people (assertion skills, listening skills, and negotiation); and increasing self-awareness (improving coping skills, problem solving and insight therapy). Outcomes of these programmes were assessed using standardised psychological self-report measures and a job performance measure (Kagan *et al.*, 1995). All three of the programmes were effective in the management of stress in both the short and long term (two years following the intervention). The self-awareness package was particularly effective in the long term.

Within the health service there have been a number of studies evaluating stress management interventions. For example, one study compared a standard SMT to training in innovation (Bunce and West, 1996). The latter intervention used group discussion to generate new and innovative ways to manage work stressors, and was based on a model of innovation (West and Farr, 1989). Although staff showed a reduction in tension experienced at work following both programmes, only staff who attended the SMT showed a general reduction in stress levels. Another study looked at training skills to improve social support and participation in decision making, thereby increasing coping resources at work (Heaney *et al.*, 1995). This study used Karasek's (1979) model of stress which proposes that people can help reduce stress when they experience an increase in workload if they are given the freedom to make more work-related decisions and have adequate levels of social support. In the health service work, overload, role conflict and interpersonal conflict have often been identified as stressors (Wall *et al.*, 1997; Firth-Cozens, 1987). The intervention by Heaney *et al.* (1995) had some positive effect on participants' ratings of supportive feedback on the job and confidence in their ability to cope with work stress, although little effect on psychological well-being. One exception to these findings was for staff intending to leave their jobs; these staff showed improvement in their well-being following the intervention. As the study was designed to enhance coping resources, it is perhaps not surprising that there was no immediate effect on mental health. Unfortunately, no long-term follow up was conducted, so it is not possible to say if the intervention did provide workers with resources to cope better with new stressors. However, the study is important because the intervention was theory based.

Another interesting study evaluated a five-week group intervention for staff working with learning disability clients (Van Dierendonck *et al.*, 1998). The intervention was based on equity theory, with the aim of reducing burnout among staff, by reducing staff perceptions of inequity in their relationship with the organisation and their relationships with clients, through improving the congruence between staffs' needs, motives and capacities and the organisation's demands and provisions. Levels of burnout decreased and sense of personal accomplishment increased in the experimental group (who received the intervention) compared to a control group within the same organisation as the experimental group and compared to a control group in another comparable organisation (neither of whom received the intervention). These improvements were maintained six months and one year following the intervention. In addition, independent, organisational-level criteria of change were used to assess the impact of the intervention. Organisationally held records of absence showed a reduction in absence taken by staff in the experimental, but not the control groups.

WORKSITE COUNSELLING

Worksite counselling includes a whole variety of methods aimed at helping individuals to cope more effectively with stress. A general framework, that can usually be used to describe most counselling procedures, is a trusting relationship between the counsellor and employee, where discussion about the client's problems will bring about resolution and change. Two broad categories of counselling or psychotherapy are offered: an "action" therapy—one that is based on cognitive and behavioural principles—or an "insight" therapy—one that is based on increasing clients' understanding of the underlying causes of distress, particularly in interpersonal relationships.

There are very few worksite counselling studies, and those that are reported suffer from the same methodological problems as studies of counselling in general. They lack specificity in describing the populations and problems being treated; there is variety and lack of specification in the treatments being offered; and heterogeneity of contrast treatments or control groups (Berridge *et al.*, 1997).

If we look at the psychotherapy literature, then there is some evidence that psychological treatments help people overcome work difficulties. However, it must be remembered that these studies are based on clinical populations—individuals who are suffering from a diagnosed psychiatric disorder—who are likely to be different to the employees who are seen by a worksite counsellor. Nevertheless, these studies are often more methodologically sound. They are usually based on either randomised controlled designs (e.g. Barkham *et al.*, 1999) or comparative outcome designs (e.g. Hardy *et al.*, 1998). In such designs, prospective clients are assessed and required to meet specified criteria before being randomly allocated to one of a number of comparative active treatments or to a control group. So, for example, in the Sheffield psychotherapy studies, clients suffering from problems at work and who were depressed, showed substantial improvements in symptoms, work behaviours and work attitudes following both cognitive-behavioural (CB) and psychodynamic-interpersonal (PI) therapies (Firth and Shapiro, 1986; Barkham and Shapiro, 1990; Firth-Cozens and Hardy, 1992). The Second Sheffield Psychotherapy Project found the CB therapy to be more effective than the PI therapy in improving work-based problems (Hardy *et al.*, 1998). Two case studies from these projects (Firth, 1985; Parry *et al.*, 1986) give a flavour of how psychotherapeutic interventions can help change individuals' perceptions about themselves and their work. However, these studies are limited in considering the value of worksite counselling because they were not conducted at the workplace, dealt with a more severe population, and did not take independent measures of work performance.

There are very few studies that assess the impact of worksite counselling. The Post Office study (Allison *et al.*, 1987) is an exception to this, and is frequently reported as evidence for the value of worksite counselling. Participants who obtained counselling showed a reduction in psychological symptomatology and reported sickness absence, compared to a control group who were matched to the counselling group on demographics (such as age, sex and grade within the organisation), but not on levels of distress, the primary target of counselling. This limits the value of the comparison group as they were more psychologically healthy than the intervention group prior to the intervention. Other studies of worksite counselling have generally found improvements in mental health, but not job satisfaction or other organisational measures (Berridge *et al.*, 1997; Shapiro *et al.*, 1993). An exception to this is the Second Sheffield Psychotherapy Project where clients were significantly more positive about aspects of their work after psychotherapy, although change in job attitudes was not as great as the change in symptomatology (Firth-Cozens and Hardy, 1992).

Counselling services are often offered within the context of employee assistance programmes (EAPs). EAPs may also provide financial and other advice services, plus specific programmes for alcohol or weight problems. Evaluations of EAPs are generally made across the whole service rather than individual components, and tend to be based on economic criteria: often the main purpose of the evaluation is to show to an organisation that such programmes are cost-effective. In addition to the methodological problems already described about counselling studies, EAP evaluations tend to be conducted by the company offering the service, who have an investment in showing the effectiveness of their work.

LIMITATIONS OF THE RESEARCH ON PSYCHOTHERAPEUTIC INTERVENTIONS

We now return to the three issues set out in the introduction. Most discussions of occupational stress incorporate at least two levels of outcome: those that affect the individual and those that affect the organisation. Even when looking at outcomes at the individual level, should psychotherapeutic interventions aim to reduce psychological symptomatology, or job dissatisfactions and organisational measures, or all three? We have seen that the evidence is still slim that SMT programmes and counselling interventions have an impact on work or organisational factors. If these are not the targets for such interventions, what remains distinctive about worksite counselling as opposed to general counselling? This is not to say that there is no place for psychotherapeutic interventions within organisations, but that far greater clarity in the procedures, mechanisms and targets for change are needed. In addition, a greater collaboration between clinical or counselling practitioners, organisational practitioners and researchers must be encouraged, so that new focused interventions can be developed and compared.

SUMMARY AND RECOMMENDATIONS

In summary, there is some evidence that counselling and SMTs have some impact on individual symptomatology. However, much of research on psychotherapeutic interventions for worksite stress is poor. If, in the first instance, we consider the development of psychotherapeutic interventions from a clinical perspective, then there are available research models that describe the development and validation of psychological interventions. For example, Linehan (1997) presents a three-stage model, which could be useful to plan research in the area. At the first stage, termed "development", an intervention is generated and specified, then standardised using pilot tests of the efficacy (testing the value of an intervention under optimal conditions). The second stage is termed "validation" and comprises further tests of efficacy, research into understanding how the intervention works (mechanisms of action) and the utility of the intervention. The final stage is termed "dissemination" and comprises service development, programme evaluation and tests of effectiveness (testing the value of an intervention in everyday actual practice). These three stages broadly represent a continuum, such that as an intervention becomes more developed, more stages in the continuum should be satisfied. Progress through each stage should feed back into the development of the intervention.

We have seen that very little sound research at the first and second stages has been conducted for worksite interventions. The implication for the third stage is self-evident. It needs to be emphasised that to conduct adequate studies of effectiveness, basic research of intervention development and rigorous studies of efficacy should first be completed. Having established that an intervention is efficacious under optimum conditions, it then needs to be established that the same intervention (together with the necessary modifications) is effective in field and applied settings— that is, when delivered as a service. The principle here is to achieve best practice derived from a robust "evidence-based" position. However, as stated earlier, the evidence base for stress management and counselling is not robust. To date, no systematic review has been carried out on SMT, and only one has been carried out specifically on counselling (in primary care) with the findings suggesting only a marginal advantage to counselling over standard GP interventions (Rowland, in preparation).

Within such a model of evidence-based practice, both SMT and counselling are seriously lacking, like the majority of other health care interventions. This has arisen in part because both SMT and counselling programmes within the work setting have developed in a rather ad hoc fashion. It has also arisen because there has been a lack of focus on the quality of interventions: McLeod (1995) calculated the number of specific outcome studies reported in two UK journals (*British Journal of Guidance and Counselling* and *Quarterly Journal of Counselling*) and one US journal (*Journal of Counseling Psychology*) over two successive years (1993–4) and found that just 6.7% of reports included a focus on the actual quality of the intervention. To establish both the efficacy and effectiveness of an intervention, quality issues are paramount.

In addition, intervention studies need to show meaningful change in client functioning rather than purely pre-post statistical change (Evans *et al.*, 1998). However, it seems likely that effect sizes will be "small" (i.e. in the region of 0.20), making it even more important that studies of work-based interventions define the specific change that is being targeted. There are also important methodological implications in that seeking such small effects will require large sample sizes. In terms of populations at work, large samples may not be difficult to achieve but they also carry with them the increased probability of obtaining a statistically significant result that is, psychologically, relatively unimportant; hence, the need to pursue more meaningful ways of interpreting data.

This has important implications, since using measures derived from other settings may not be sufficiently sensitive to register important changes obtained in work settings. Future requirements within the domain of interventions for work stress include a comprehensive database of norms to be able to determine whether a particular intervention has met an agreed standard.

As can be seen from this three-stage developmental model, the "quality" of the service provision to workers is a function of theoretical models of psychological interventions being validated under optimum conditions and then adapted and modified to be effective in the field together with such implementation processes being audited and outcomes monitored. If outcomes do not approximate those obtained under optimum conditions, but auditing the implementation shows a lack of adherence to protocols, then this can be rectified. If the outcomes are similarly poor even though appropriate implementation processes have been adhered to, then the theoretical models underpinning the psychological interventions need to be reviewed. Such an iterative process will then advance the delivery of a strong evidence base for psychotherapeutic interventions for work stress.

Other recommendations for future service development have been implicit in the foregoing review. They span two broad areas. First, services need to be more focused:

1. What works for whom in what circumstances? This has implications for the training and setting up of counselling services. Generic counselling to all comers of a service that aims to help all problems is probably neither an effective nor an efficient way to run a worksite counselling service.
2. It is possible that the more generic counselling skills are better utilised by line managers for managing the day-to-day hassles and difficulties experienced by staff. Managerial support and performance feedback are valued by staff and have been shown to be related to change in levels of stress.
3. More problematic, long-lasting difficulties are perhaps more appropriately dealt with by counsellors, where changing work conditions may be insufficient to help someone who is extremely distressed or suffers from very low self-esteem.

Second, there needs to be more applied, good evaluative research and audit.

4. However, this can best be progressed through adopting a robust model that sets out the interrelationships between theoretical models, efficacy research and practice, together with the monitoring function of audit.

5. Evaluation, in whatever form it takes, needs to be integrated within practice as opposed to "added on". In this way, it becomes "owned" by the respective parties.

REFERENCES

Allison, T., Cooper, C.L. and Reynolds, P. (1987). Stress counselling in the workplace—The Post Office experience. *The Psychologist*, **12**, 384–388.

Auerbach, S.M. (1989). Stress management and coping research in the health care setting: an overview of methodological commentary. *Journal of Consulting and Clinical Psychology*, **57**, 388–395.

Barkham, M. and Shapiro, D.A. (1990). Brief psychotherapeutic interventions for job-related distress: a pilot of prescriptive and exploratory therapy. *Counselling Psychology Review*, **3**, 133–147.

Barkham, M., Shapiro, D.A., Hardy, G.E. and Rees, A. (1999). Psychotherapy in two-plus-one sessions: outcomes of a randomized controlled trial of cognitive-behavioral and psychodynamic-interpersonal therapy for subsyndromal depression. *Journal of Consulting and Clinical Psychology*, **67**, 201–211.

Beehr, T.A. and O'Hara, K. (1987). Methodological designs for the evaluation of occupational stress interventions. In S.V. Cooper and C.L. Cooper (Eds) *Stress and Health: Issues in Research Methodology*. Chichester: Wiley.

Berridge, J. and Cooper, C. (1993). Stress and coping in US organizations: the role of the Employee Assistance Programme. *Work and Stress*, **7**, 89–102.

Berridge, J., Cooper, C.L. and Highley-Marchington, C. (1997). *Employee Assistance Programmes and Workplace Counselling*. Chichester: Wiley.

Bunce, D. and West, M.A. (1996). Stress management and innovation at work. *Human Relations*, **49**, 209–232.

Caplan, R.D., Cobb, S., French, J.R.P., Van Harrison, R.V. amd Pinneau, S. R. (1975). *Job Demands and Worker Health*. Washington DC: US Department of Health, Education and Welfare.

Cooper, C.L. and Cartwright, S. (1994). Healthy mind; healthy organization—a proactive approach to occupational stress. *Human Relations*, **47**, 455–471.

Cooper, C.L. and Sadri, G. (1991). The impact of stress counselling at work. *Journal of Social Behavior and Personality*, **6**, 411–423.

Depue, R.A. and Monroe, S.M. (1988). Conceptualization and measurement of human disorder in life stress research: the problem of chronic disturbance. *Psychological Bulletin*, **99**, 36–51.

Elkin, I., Shea, M.T., Watkins, J.T., Imber, S.D., Sotsky, S., Collins, J.F., Glass, D.R., Pilkonis, P.A., Leber, W.R., Docherty, J.P., Fiester, S.J. and Parloff, M.B. (1989). National Institute of Mental Health Treatment of Depression Collaborative Research Program: general effectiveness of treatments. *Archives of General Psychiatry*, **46**, 971–982.

Evans, C., Margison, F. and Barkham, M. (1998). The contribution of reliable and clinically significant change methods to evidence-based mental health. *Evidence-Based Mental Health*, **1**, 70–72.

Everly, S.E. (1989). *A Clinical Guide to the Treatment of the Human Stress Response*. New York: Plenum.

Firth, J.A. (1985). Personal meanings of occupational stress: cases from the clinic. *Journal of Occupational Psychology*, **58**, 139–148.

Firth-Cozens, J. (1987). Emotional distress in junior house officers. *British Medical Journal*, **295**, 533–536.

Firth-Cozens, J. and Hardy, G.E. (1992). Occupational stress, clinical treatment and changes in job perceptions. *Journal of Occupational and Organizational Psychology*, **65**, 81–88.

Firth, J.A. and Shapiro, D.A. (1986). An evaluation of psychotherapy for job-related distress. *Journal of Occupational Psychology*, **59**, 111–119.

Fisher, S. (1986). *Stress and Strategy*. London: Lawrence Erlbaum Associates.

Ganster, D.C., Mayes, B.T., Sime, W.E. and Tharp, G.D. (1982). Managing organizational stress: a field experiment. *Journal of Applied Psychology*, **76**, 533–542.

Hardy, G.E., Reynolds, S., Shapiro, D.A. and Barkham, M. (1998). The comparison of cognitive-behavioural with psychodynamic-interpersonal therapy for the treatment of work difficulties associated with depression. Unpublished manuscript. University of Leeds.

Heaney, C.A., Price, R.H. and Refferty, J. (1995). Increasing coping resources at work: a field experiment to increase social support, improve team functioning, and enhance employee mental health. *Journal of Organizational Behavior*, **16**, 335–352.

Ivancevich, J.M., Matteson, M.T., Freedman, S.M. and Phillips, J.S. (1990). Worksite stress management interventions. *American Psychologist*, **45**, 252–261.

Jones, K.R., DeBaca, B.N., Steffy, B.D., Fay, L.M., Kuntz, L.K. and Wuebker, L.J. (1988). Stress and medical malpractice: organizational risk assessment and intervention. *Journal of Applied Psychology*, **73**, 727–735.

Kagan, N.I., Kagan, H. and Watson, M.G. (1995). Stress reduction in the workplace: the effectiveness of psychoeducational programs. *Journal of Counseling Psychology*, **42**, 71–78.

Karasek, R.A. (1979). Job demands, job decisions latitude and mental strain: implications for job redesign. *Administrative Science Quarterly*, **24**, 285–308.

Kobasa, S.C., Maddi, S.R. and Kahn, S. (1982). Hardiness and health: a prospective study. *Journal of Personality and Social Psychology*, **42**, 168–177.

Linehan, M. (1997). Treatment development, validation and dissemination: thoughts from the trenches. Keynote address, *13th Annual Meeting of the Society for Psychotherapy Research, Ravenscar, UK*.

McLeod, J. (1995). Evaluating the effectiveness of counselling. What we don't know. *Changes*, **13**, 192–200.

Mintz, J., Mintz, L.M., Arruda, M.J. and Hwang, S.S. (1992). Treatments of depression and the functional capacity to work. *Archives of General Psychiatry*, **49**, 761–768.

Murphy, L.R. (1996). Stress management in work settings: a critical review. *American Journal of Health Promotions*, **11**, 112–135.

Parry, G., Shapiro, D. A. and Firth, J. A. (1986). The case of the anxious executive: a study from the research clinic. *British Journal of Medical Psychology*, **59**, 221–233.

Reynolds, S. and Shapiro, D. A. (1991). Stress reduction in transition: conceptual problems in the design, implementation, and evaluation of worksite stress management interventions. *Human Relations*, **44**, 717–733.

Rosenman, R.H. and Chesney, M.A. (1985). Type A behavior and coronary heart disease: a review of theory and findings. In P.B. Defares (Ed.) *Stress and Anxiety*, Vol. 9. Washington: Hemisphere Publishing Corp.

Roth, A. and Fonagy. P. (1996). *What Works for Whom? A Critical Review of Psychotherapy Research*. New York: Guilford Press.

Rowland, N. (in preparation). Review of counselling in primary care.

Sallis, J.F., Trevorrow, T.R., Johnson, C.C., Hovell, M.F. and Kaplan, R.M. (1987). Worksite stress management: a comparison of programmes. *Psychology and Health*, **1**, 237–255.

Shapiro, D.A., Cheesman, M. and Wall, T.D. (1993). Secondary prevention— Review of counselling and EAPs. *SAPU Memo No. 1401*. University of Sheffield.

Van Dierendonck, D., Schaufeli, W.B. and Buunk, B.P. (1998). The evaluation of an individual burnout intervention program: the role of inequity and social support. *Journal of Applied Psychology*, **83**, 392–407.

Wall, T.D., Bolden, R.I., Borrill, C.S., Carter, A., Hardy, G.E., Haynes, C., Rick, J., Shapiro, D.A. and West, M.A. (1997). Minor psychiatric disorder in NHS trust staff: occupational and gender differences. *British Journal of Psychiatry*, **171**, 519–523.

West, M.A. and Farr, J. (1989). Innovation at work: psychological perspectives. *Social Behavior*, **4**, 15–30.

INDEX

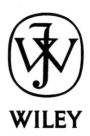